The Rise and Fall of High Fructose Corn Syrup and Fibromyalgia

The Rise and Fall of High Fructose Corn Syrup and Fibromyalgia

*Ending Fibromyalgia Without
Drugs or Violence*

Janice Lorigan

authorHOUSE®

AuthorHouse™
1663 Liberty Drive
Bloomington, IN 47403
www.authorhouse.com
Phone: 1-800-839-8640

The advice contained in this book should be used only with the approval of your own physician. Consult with a medical doctor for all health problems, including fibromyalgia.

First published by AuthorHouse   06/20/2011

ISBN: 978-1-4634-0786-5 (sc)
ISBN: 978-1-4634-0785-8 (dj)
ISBN: 978-1-4634-1980-6 (ebk)

Library of Congress Control Number: 2011909137

Printed in the United States of America

This book is printed on acid-free paper.

DEDICATION: With love to Matt, Amber, Nando and
all the Finleys, especially Jim

"The word is so full of a number of things, I'm sure we
should all
Be as happy as Kings"

Robert Louis Stevenson

CONTENTS

Introduction 1

One　　　　What Fibromyalgia Is And What It Is Not 7

Two　　　　Fibromyalgia Recovery Plans 13

Three　　　Birth And Growth Of Fibromyalgia 17

Four　　　　Alternative Treatments For Fibromyalgia...................22

Five　　　　The Princeton Study 32

Six　　　　　The Manufacture Of High Fructose Corn Syrup 41

Seven　　　Metabolism And Xenobiotics 46

Eight　　　　Causes Of Fibromyalgia 51

Nine　　　　From Upton Sinclair To Xenobiotics 57

Ten　　　　　Fascia, Pain, And The Central Nervous System 71

Eleven　　　Fatigue And Energy......................................76

Twelve　　　Under The Radar 79

Thirteen　　Fibromyalgia, Science, And Research 84

Fourteen　　Invisible To The Naked Eye 95

Fifteen　　　My Recovery Story......................................101

Sixteen　　　Good Health 109

Seventeen　Happy Ending...119

INTRODUCTION

The Rise and Fall of High Fructose Corn Syrup and Fibromyalgia include two recovery plans—one of which will end fibromyalgia pain and other fibromyalgia symptoms for almost everyone. The first plan is easy to follow and will end most fibromyalgia symptoms for many. The second plan may be the best plan for those whose fibromyalgia problems are nearly constant. In addition to alleviating fibromyalgia symptoms, the second plan contributes to overall health and well-being. Neither plan will cause negative side effects. There are no pills to swallow, and there is nothing to buy or order. You will be given the knowledge and power to end fibromyalgia symptoms and enhance overall health.

The most important messages contained in this book are those that will help you live a good life with restored energy and without the reoccurring cycle of pain and misery. Relief for your own pain, suffering, and fatigue is most likely the reason you have decided to read the book. A few of the chapters are technical, and one is personal. My struggle began in 1976 with multiple symptoms of unexplained origin and embarrassment for absences from work for which I had no standard medical excuses. I document many of the holistic and traditional interventions that gave little to no relief. I have been recovered since the spring of 2007.

For emphasis, a separate chapter explains the hidden nature of the biochemical dynamics of high fructose corn syrup. In short, almost everyone has been "fooled" for quite a long time. It is unusual to find any other ingredient that is this hidden to this great of a degree. High fructose corn syrup has avoided scrutiny of scientists. It has circumvented notice of those suffering with fibromyalgia. One reason the causal relationship continues without being noticed, even by those with fibromyalgia, is that the cause and effect relationship has a significant period of delay. Unlike the nearly instant reaction speed of food allergies, the impact of high fructose corn syrup usually strikes two to four days after ingestion. This long lull between the consumption of high fructose corn syrup and the unwelcome symptoms masks the cause and effect relationship.

The materials of the book are organized to answer questions regarding causes and recovery. Be sure to read the chapter about the important 2010 Princeton study on high fructose corn syrup.

The information combined from several chapters describes the relationship of the body's communication system and metabolism. Blood circulates throughout the body in approximately one minute. Pain receptors in the skin signal "ouch" to the brain in less than a second. Almost everything that is taken into the body affects all parts of the body, in varying degrees. All the effects of metabolism take some time, but communication in the body is rapid.

Residues from drugs, natural or prescription medications, and Vitamin D all make their way into teeth, hair, nails, the bloodstream, and organs. All ingredients contained in food and beverages have the potential to affect the body in either a positive or negative way. Providing answers and explanations for those suffering with fibromyalgia to questions such as "What has happened to me?" and "Why?" require some technical information regarding internal biochemical functions.

The most difficult task for me has been to provide adequate and pertinent information on somewhat complex subjects in a clear, explicit manner. Hopefully, this book represents a generous amount of clarity, fairness, and honesty.

Chemicals exist everywhere. Some are beneficial to humans; and some, are not. Xenobiotics are substances that are foreign to humans. Several man-made xenobiotics and a portion of high fructose corn syrup with denatured DNA and unbound molecules are strongly correlated with fibromyalgia. Molecules of those noxious substances work against efficient metabolic functions and often cause internal disruption.

High fructose corn syrup was introduced to the United States in the early 1970s. In 1976, generous amounts were infused into American beverages and processed food products. A few years later unfamiliar symptoms began to be reported to doctors and clinicians in the United States. Complaints of the unusual set of symptoms revealed a new and baffling illness. For years, many doctors dismissed the complaints as "neurotic" or "psychogenic" because the total set of complaints didn't fall into any established medical model. Fibromyalgia was given its name sometime in the 1980s, and the condition began to be accepted as "real" by some a few years later. As the number of food products with high fructose corn syrup grew—The adjective "exponentially" is not an exaggeration here—so did the growing numbers of people diagnosed with fibromyalgia.

Currently, there is a tremendous push by manufacturers and representatives of the Corn Refiners Association to convince the FDA to allow the name "corn sugar" to be used in public messages and on ingredient labels of food products—in essence, to replace the words "high fructose corn syrup." These lobbyists and marketing reps are backed by agri-business which reaps profits annually in the multi-billions. They have long-standing relationships with the FDA, and they are powerful. As a point of comparison, some may recall the intense, lengthy fight waged by the tobacco industry against putting warnings on the side of cigarette packages.

If you begin to see or hear the new name "corn sugar," you will know that the lobbyists prevailed, and the name "high fructose corn syrup" will gradually disappear. If marketing and public relations representatives of agri-business succeed with this deception, tell your friends and neighbors and remind yourself that CORN SUGAR IS HIGH FRUCTOSE CORN SYRUP.

Whether it is called "corn sugar" or "high fructose corn syrup," the chemical bonds have been broken in the manufacturing process. The basic DNA has been denatured, and the free molecules have the potential to enter the bloodstream and cause havoc in the central nervous system and metabolism. The unbound molecules of high fructose corn syrup allow for a type of free radical, reactive carbonyls, to circulate throughout the body.

You have the power to make good choices. Mom's quote seems appropriate now, "A word to the wise is sufficient."
To days blessed with health and joy,

Janice Lorigan
April 27, 2011

Chapter One

What Fibromyalgia Is and What It Is Not

Fibromyalgia is a biochemical disorder characterized by widespread pain, fatigue, and stiffness in the connective tissue. Other symptoms include achiness, irritable bowel and spastic bladder, headaches, depression or catastrophic thinking, increased sensitivity to pain, and unrefreshing or disturbed sleep. The term "fibromyalgia" means pain in the fibrous (connective) tissue.

The symptoms of fibromyalgia are intermittent or cyclical. Some describe the worst symptoms as changing in intensity, or "waxing and waning." The discomfort of fibromyalgia is often significant and debilitating.

Fibromyalgia is a biochemical disorder that stems from unbound molecules circulating in the bloodstream reaching the central nervous system and soft tissue and the fascia. The dysfunction is caused by chemicals from the environment that confound and stall metabolic processes at the cellular level. These synthetic chemicals are referred to as xenobiotics (foreign). Typically, the chemical molecules from the environment are transported into the body as very small subparts of food and beverages. However, there are some toxic particles in the air, and they can be breathed into the body.

Fibromyalgia falls short of the strictest definitions of "disease". A section of the Food and Drug Administration guidelines defines disease as something that causes damage to the system of the body, causing improper functioning, or damage to an organ or body part or causing a health status that leads to dysfunction (cardiovascular disease, for example.) The FDA excludes conditions that are caused by the lack of important nutrients (examples given in the guidelines are pellagra and scurvy).

As far as we know, fibromyalgia does not permanently damage any tissue or organ in the body. The FDA's definition of "dysfunction" seems to imply a state of dysfunction for a long period of time or over a life-time. The dysfunction is usually located in a specific body part or organ. Fibromyalgia metabolic dysfunction is not constant, cannot be observed, and cannot be measured, at this point.

There is no evidence of a causal relationship with viruses or bacteria in cases of fibromyalgia. Fibromyalgia is not caused by a virus, and it is not contagious. Like rheumatism, it is often referred to as a "condition." Some may consider fibromyalgia as a type of rheumatism. However, fibromyalgia includes a broader range of symptoms than those of rheumatism. Like rheumatism, fibromyalgia is not considered by medical personnel to be a disease. Some believe that fibromyalgia is fibrosistis. However, the definitions of fibrosistis do not include chronic fatigue and other typical fibromyalgia problems such as irritable bowel and un-refreshing sleep.

One distinction between fibromyalgia and many other ailments is the phenomena of stiff and inflexible fascia around the body's back, upper torso, neck and head. The fascia is a stretchy substance that lies beneath the skin and lies over muscles and organs. The fascia of the body is fibroelastic, meaning the fascia has properties like fibers and has also an elastic quality. For a part of a fibromyalgia bout, the elastic part of the fascia is shortened or temporarily looses its elastic quality. It becomes difficult to feel flexible and comfortable while that phenomena is occurring. Many with fibromyalgia enjoy back and neck massages or even rubbing the middle of their backs against available door jambs on uncomfortable days.

It has been reported that the term "fibromyalgia" was coined in the early 1980s. Most people had never heard the term until the mid 1980s, or later. Before 1970, no medical dictionaries, textbooks, medical encyclopedias, or literature included the word "fibromyalgia." Fibromyalgia existed in the American population approximately eight or nine years before the condition was recognized as a legitimate biological problem.

No book with a publication date earlier than 1970 includes the word "fibromyalgia". Finding legitimacy and being accepted as "real" took quite a few years. Prior to 1985, most doctors did not recognize the unique set of symptoms. After lupus, arthritis, and other problems were ruled out, some doctors assumed that the best recourse might be exercise, psychotherapy, and/or anti-depressants.

For a while medical personnel were perplexed by the complaints of pain because of the lack of observable injuries to the body, lack of evidence of an infectious disease, and lack of evidence of cancer or organ malfunction. Some with fibromyalgia look healthy and even robust. In the 1980s, no causes had been identified. Many doctors and others assumed that the root of the problem was psychogenic or psychosomatic in origin.

In some ways, fibromyalgia seems related to metabolic disorders. Both conditions are believed to spring from problems with enzymes (or lack of them) or xenobiotics in the endocrine system of the body. However, some characteristics of fibromyalgia do not apply to metabolic disorders. Some metabolic disorders have strong genetic components. Tay-Sachs is an example of a metabolic disorder with a genetic component. Some metabolic disorders result, in part, from organ dysfunction or damage. (Examples include pancreatic dysfunction associated with diabetes or liver impairment in fatty liver disease.) The intermittent nature of fibromyalgia and its lack of association with high blood presssure and higher levels of sugar in the blood fall outside the understanding of metabolic syndrome, syndrome X. Its lack of a genetic component is uncharacteristic of a metabolic disorder.

SOME COMMON MEDICAL CLASSIFICATIONS

Autoimmune disorders   Infectious Diseases
Organ malfunction or failure   Cancer
Allergies   Food Intolerance
Digestive disorders   Metabolic disorders
Asthma and lung disorders   Cardiovascular disorders
Poisoning and environmental disorders
Disorders of the brain and inflammation of the spinal column
Paralysis
Autism
Strokes

Fibromyalgia does not fully match any of the above established medical classifications. Fibromyalgia is relatively new, and its lack of conformity to the above models added confusion for researchers and others, for some time.

Fibromyalgia comes close to merging two of the above disorders—(1) metabolic disorders and (2) poisoning and environmental disorders. Later chapters will explain this position a little more fully.

Fibromyalgia does not have "disease" characteristics. It is not caused by a virus, bacteria, or organ failure. There is no increase in the number of white blood cells (cells that are generated to fight infections). Usually, body temperature and pulse remain in normal ranges. Bouts of fibromyalgia are cyclical, and the pain and very low energy that occur parallel the struggle of metabolism to expel toxins or poisons from the body. Fibromyalgia does not fall into the medical classification of disease. "Disorder," "syndrome," or "condition" are the commonly used words in definitions.

To many of you, recovering quickly is of greater importance than understanding much of the above. I will provide recovery plans in the following chapter that will begin your recovery from fibromyalgia. You can begin right away to prevent future bouts of this dreadful condition. It isn't reasonable to expect significant results in the first two weeks. In less than four weeks, you will notice considerable improvement. At the conclusion of four months—relief from chronic pain, a feeling of control, and a renewed belief in "cures."

CHAPTER TWO

FIBROMYALGIA RECOVERY PLANS

The fibromyalgia recovery plans on the following pages detail specific guidelines to stop fibromyalgia symptoms by minimizing or blocking the root causes of fibromyalgia.

PLAN A

Many will find success with Plan A. It is simple because its sole purpose is to make certain that no high fructose corn syrup enters your body.

Important: The deleterious effects of high fructose corn syrup begin to be felt, usually, between two and four days after ingestion. Recovery progress may take two or more weeks before major progress is noticed.

1. Read all ingredient labels prior to purchasing. Exclude any products that contain high fructose corn syrup. (Old-time corn syrup is fine.)

2. Ask at restaurants and fast food establishments if buns, barbeque sauce, salad dressing, etc. contain high fructose corn syrup. If there is a good chance that something does contain high fructose corn syrup (example, hot dog bun at a drive-through fast food restaurant), err on the side of caution.

3. Cook and prepare foods that are completely free of high fructose corn syrup.

4. Use extra caution with beverages. Currently, many sweetened beverages and fruit drinks contain high fructose corn syrup.

** Any and all products with labels saying "organic" are completely free of high fructose corn syrup (HFCS).

PLAN B

Those with the most chronic and almost everyday symptoms of fibromyalgia may need stricter dietary guidelines. Plan B is designed to eliminate high fructose corn syrup, monosodium glutamate (MSG), aspartame, and several man-made chemicals from the diet. In addition, following the guidelines of Plan B will also minimize the amount of consumption of residue from pesticides and herbicides, and reduce the amount of some chemicals often contained in water, such as hexachlorophene (chromium 6) and arsenic.

1. Eat only processed foods that are labeled "organic".

2. Carefully wash all fruits and vegetables before eating.

3. Be careful of sauces, breading, and spices that are added to meat, fish, or poultry. Reject any foods or spices with additives that contain high fructose corn syrup, monosodium glutamate (MSG), or aspartame.

4. Do not eat bacon, wieners, sausages or cold cuts made with processed meats.

5. Drink only beverages that do not contain additives or high fructose corn syrup. Usually the safest beverages are organic juice, coffee, unsweetened teas, and filtered water.

6. Be very selective of food choices at restaurants, and inquire about ingredients in products such as salad dressings, barbeque sauce, pies and desserts, muffins, marinara sauces, and all bread products.

7. When cooking use the healthiest spices, such as cinnamon, pepper, turmeric, coriander, and curry and chili powders. Wash herbs carefully. Do not use flavor enhancers or meat rubs that contain monosodium glutamate.

8. When possible drink filtered water or water from a clean spring source. (Some bottled waters may meet that requirement.)

Plan A is easier. However, Plan B eliminates many toxins and can contribute more to overall health.

CHAPTER THREE

BIRTH AND GROWTH OF FIBROMYALGIA

Current estimates of the number of Americans who have been diagnosed with fibromyalgia range from three percent to five percent of the total population (that translates to millions of Americans). There was no fibromyalgia prior to 1970. Complaints of a unique set of symptoms chiefly characterized by complaints of all-over, unexplained pain began to reach the medical world in the 1970's. Medical doctors, scientists, clinicians, and lay persons all were perplexed and baffled for years after hearing accounts of unrelenting pain, fatigue, stiffness, and a general malaise. Initially some of the symptoms of fibromayalgia would partially fit labels of fibrosistis, rheumatism, arthritis, food sensitivity, or neurosis. However, none of those afflictions encompassed all the fibromyalgia symptoms; and therefore, there was no thorough, accurate fit.

Later in the 1970s or early 1980s, the medical world began to see the growing number of common reports as indicative of a real bio-chemical disorder. However, there were no answers from medical schools, textbooks, or journals. A few doctors clung to the idea that overall organic or biochemical causes were lacking. Therefore, some doctors recommended antidepressants or talk therapies to patients.

In the 1980s in North America someone coined the term "fibromyalgia." It began to be recognized as a distinct real medical problem, although it was still not understood or recognized by many. The common description of fibromyalgia became "fibromyalgia syndrome."

Reports of fibromyalgia became more and more frequent over much of the United States and Canada. The number of people diagnosed with fibromyalgia continued to grow larger each year. By the 1990s, many in the larger society began to acknowledge fibromyalgia as a legitimate condition or disorder.

No effective cures existed for the total set of fibromyalgia symptoms. The primary reason for the lack of cures is simply that, for several years, causes had not been discovered. (No cause, no cure.) To further disguise fibromyalgia and make finding causes more difficult was the phenomena of no observable symptoms. In addition, there were no common medical markers of physical distress or dysfunction, such as fever, uncommon blood measurements, evidence of infection or increase in the number of white blood cells, irregularities in the spine, tumor growth, etc. Fibromyalgia dysfunctions are rooted deep in the body at the enzymatic and cellular level, affecting even the functioning of the mitochondria in the cells. The study of mitochondria, enzymatic action and neurotransmitters in the central nervous system are relatively new scientific fields. These studies involve studying the smallest of micro particles, fluids, and chemical interactions.

Countries such as Great Britain, Australia, New Zealand, Canada and the U.S. all report growing incidences of fibromyalgia. Accounts of fibromyalgia are absent from the least industrialized parts of the world and areas that have remained rural and agrarian. The inhabitants there are cut off from grocery stores and processed foods. Of course, some of these areas are also devoid or very deficient in record—keeping making it difficult to evaluate whether or not fibromyalgia even exists there. However, I believe those insulated areas are protected from fibromyalgia and a few other newer medical conditions that have no known cures, because the inhabitants of agrarian, non-industrialized areas do not eat processed foods. In these agrarian parts of the world, reports of Parkinson's, Alzheimer's, ADD, and autism are usually rare.

Fibromyalgia developed and grew beginning in the mid 1970s, and incidence reports became more frequent in the 1980s and 1990s. At the same time fibromyalgia was growing, high fructose corn syrup was manufactured in much greater quantities and infused into many more food products. Products containing high fructose corn syrup number into the thousands.

High fructose corn syrup was infused into a few foods in the early 1970s. A smooth manufacturing process was put into use in the mid-1970s, and the use of high fructose corn syrup grew exponentially throughout the 1970s, 1980s, and 1990s. Thousands of foods and beverages containing high fructose corn syrup were manufactured and marketed, especially between 1976 and 2007. Some manufacturers in the mid 2000s replaced HFCS with beet or cane sugar, artificial sweeteners, molasses, maple syrup, or honey. Currently, there is a trend to discontinue high fructose corn syrup as an ingredient. Now, many manufacturers have quietly removed it from their processed food formulae. Some manufacturers choose to print "No High Fructose Corn Syrup" on the label to attract more health-conscious consumers.

Fibromyalgia symptoms are not common in children. There are significant differences in metabolic functioning of a child of eight and an adult who is thirty-seven or forty-nine. Age of first diagnosis is generally after age twenty. It affects all races and ethnicities. The most striking difference is that many more females than males have a fibromyalgia diagnosis. Some estimate that eighty to ninety percent of all fibromyalgia sufferers are female.

However, males also develop fibromyalgia, as do some teenagers.

It is not rare to have conditions or diseases that affect the sexes differently. Autism, schizophrenia, and some behavioral disorders affect more males than females. Lupus, metabolic syndrome, and fibromyalgia affect more females than males. Early on, research was focused on hormonal differences between those with a fibromyalgia diagnosis and those who were free of the affliction. No significant hormone level differences were found between those with fibromyalgia and those without.

High fructose corn syrup and fibromyalgia reports nearly parallel each other in quantity and growth during the years of 1976 through 2006. Fibromyalgia is a biochemical condition with causes that are linked with food additives and processed food products. Fibromyalgia and high fructose corn syrup appear to have a much greater connection than just a coincidental surge in the same time period.

Chapter Four

ALTERNATIVE TREATMENTS FOR FIBROMYALGIA

The recovery methods outlined in THE RISE AND FALL OF HIGH FRUCTOSE CORN SYRUP AND FIBROMYALGIA are not the only treatments. Also, the treatments discussed in this chapter do not include every available fibromyalgia treatment. The included treatments are those most commonly used.

On medical websites and in published materials, fibromyalgia has a definition that follows with words to this effect, " . . . there is no cure." I believe that statement is false (based on my experience and the reports of others). Absolute statements about "no cure" are false and very misleading. It would be accurate and fair to say, "cures are in the early stage of development" or "no one cure is completely accepted in the scientific community at this point."

There are cures for nearly everything at some point. The development of cures takes time. Research, experimentation, controls, replication of successful experiments, documentation, and communication all contribute to a lengthy process. Fibromyalgia presents a greater challenge than challenges presented by several other medical issues for reasons that are discussed in later chapters. At first, fibromyalgia was not recognized as a biochemical disorder, but was rather excused as a psychosomatic problem. Specific causes have been very slow to surface. (Without identification of cause or causes, total resolution of any problem is extremely difficult. Identification of the specific cause is critical to all problem solving.) In addition, major corporations have huge fiduciary interests in the long-term treatment of the symptoms of fibromyalgia. The focus of pharmaceutical companies is discovering, manufacturing and marketing products for treatments of SYMPTOMS only. An effective cure shortens or diminishes the time needed for their product, and effective cures can threaten their "bottom line." Pharmaceutical companies thrive on symptom treatment, and there are few incentives to concentrate efforts on discovering causes and cures.

The following alternative treatments have shown varying degrees of success. Usually, a treatment is intended for only one or two specific problems of fibromyalgia, such as all-over pain or stiffness in the back and shoulders. Some of the discussed treatments require medical prescriptions, and some are considered natural.

Antidepressants

Beginning several decades ago, antidepressants were prescribed to minimize depression for people complaining of fibromyalgia and for those with general depression. Antidepressants can give a modest boost to the spirits of those with fibromyalgia. There are no reports of comprehensive relief for all fibromyalgia symptoms resulting from regular use of antidepressants.

Tai Chi, Massage, Stretching, and Acupressure

Tai Chi, massage, stretching and acupressure all have therapeutic use. However, there have been no reports of any of them preventing bouts of fibromyalgia symptoms. All four—tai chi, massage, stretching, and acupressure—have the potential to alleviate some of the tightness and misery that stem from fascia that has lost its elasticity and constricted connective tissue. These therapies have limited use for all-over pain.

Meditation and Deep Breathing

Very few are able to effectively use meditation to prevent or end fibromyalgia. However, both meditation and deep breathing can minimize some forms of pain. In addition, both deep breathing and meditation have subtle benefits for many people. Deep breathing and meditation both lead to relaxation which can defend against pain, but neither has proved to thoroughly end all fibromyalgia symptoms.

Over the Counter Products (OTC)

Those suffering with fibromyalgia give reports of limited success achieved by taking recommended doses of aspirin, ibuprofen, or naproxen sodium. Each of these common over-the-counter drugs may reduce some pain. Unfortunately, the pain of fibromyalgia is too intense to be completely eradicated. When I was suffering with bouts of fibromyalgia, aspirin was not very effective for my pain. However, aspirin seemed to help me sleep a little more soundly and deeply. Aspirin has preventive and healing qualities and has proven over time to be close to a "wonder drug."

Using a heating pad or sitting in a hot tub for a while is soothing. Others claim those maneuvers provide partial relief, at best.

Electroconvulsive Therapy (ECT)

There have been a few reports of successful pain treatment using electroconvulsive therapy. Japanese researchers at the Juntendo University School of Medicine used Visual Analog Scales (VAS) to assess pain levels before and after treatment of patients complaining of severe pain. The VAS is a system of numbering the degree of pain (from 0 to 10) through patient self-reporting. The researchers reported significant lessening of pain and improved blood flow in the thalamus portion of the brain of the subjects who underwent several sessions of electroconvulsive therapy.

Improvements have been made to electroconvulsive therapy in recent years. However, the treatment works by passing electrical currents through the brain to trigger a brief controlled seizure. ECT is more frequently used for cases of extreme depression.

The side effects of electroconvulsive therapy include confusion soon after treatment and the possibility of muscle spasms, vomiting, headaches, and nausea.

Fibromyalgia Prescription Medications

Guaifenesin is a chelating agent that was once prescribed to reduce symptoms. Chelation is a chemical acid that binds ions of metals in the body to prevent accumulation of toxic levels.

Some with fibromyalgia took guaifenesin daily for months. A lack of positive reports of guaifenesin effectiveness and the popularity of better-marketed medications have overtaken the sales and interest in guaifenesin. (Prior to fibromyalgia, guaifenesin was recognized and used as an effective expectorant in cold medications.)

Prescription medications are not expected to prevent all fibromyalgia symptoms. Most are fairly effective at reducing pain by mediating some neurotransmitters in the central nervous system. The current prescription drugs do not cure fibromyalgia, but they do reduce some of the pain by administering very powerful drugs.

Side effects are certainly the most glaring drawback to long-term, daily use of fibromyalgia prescription medications. Some medications are classified as antiepileptic drugs and can intensify depression or thoughts of suicide. Possible serious allergic reactions to fibromyalgia medications are breathing difficulties and/or swelling of the neck, throat, mouth, tongue, or face. Other possible side effects of many medications include weight gain, muscle soreness or weakness, blurry vision, swelling of feet and hands, and trouble concentrating. A few potential side effects are indicative of permanent organ damage or failure. Typically, consumers are advised to discontinue use and call their doctors immediately upon notice of severe side effects.

Legally, pharmaceutical companies are required to warn consumers of the potential undesirable effects, referred to as "common side effects" and "possible side effects." It may be awkward to list all the side effects in television commercials because the commercials would be rather lengthy. The negative side effects announced would probably take attention away from the positive, desirable characteristics of medications. Therefore, pharmaceutical representatives submit warnings along with the ads to magazines for wide distribution. Although the ads with subsequent lists and warnings are not an attractive feature of magazines, they serve to warn consumers and protect the company from potential legal action.

Organic Foods Only

There are anecdotal reports of nearly complete recovery from fibromyalgia by people who experimented with diets that included raw foods and plentiful quantities of organic food. All processed foods were excluded. The people who devoted time to this diet did so for a variety of reasons and health concerns. Recovery from fibromyalgia was an unexpected benefit for some.

There is not much documentation on these accounts. Perhaps because fibromyalgia wasn't the singular interest or primary interest of the participants. There are so many variables that are unknown, such as, were they all eating the same types of food? Did they drink filtered water? Were all types of sugar (except maybe maple syrup and honey) excluded from all foods? How many participants were in this experiment? How many in the group had been previously diagnosed with fibromyalgia? Were they eating vegetables and fruits in multiples of what the average American would eat? This was an informal study. There was no control group, and many "confounding" variables detract from the study and its results.

Although the reports are not based on legitimate science, there are still some compelling implications. I find the reports of success believable. If all the participants ate no processed foods or seasoned foods and drank nothing but water or drinks considered organic, then they consumed no high fructose corn syrup, no monosodium glutamate, no aspartame, no sorbitol, no sucralose, no disodium guanylate, no sodium aluminum phosphate, etc., etc.

These anecdotal reports of the organic food experiments are inferior sources of data. However, success with this kind of diet does seem very possible. (You may have realized that if drinking filtered water and thoroughly washing all fruits and vegetables had been added to the organic regimen described above, it would be nearly the same treatment as Plan B of chapter two of this book.)

There are four distinctions between Plans A and B of this book and almost all other treatments:

- Plans A and B are dietary elimination plans that are believed to be related to the underlying causes. (In contrast to methods or plans that are directed at alleviating symptoms.)

- There are no known deleterious effects from either Plan A or Plan B.

- The plans of this book do not require on-going, expensive treatment protocols.

- Both plans of this book may improve overall health, in addition to knocking out fibromyalgia symptoms, on a long-term basis. Plan B may minimize facial break-outs for many because of the elimination of nearly all xenobiotics from food and ultimately their bodies.

In addition to the positives listed above, scientists now believe that high fructose corn syrup raises triglyceride levels in blood of most people. (Triglycerides is a technical term for bad fat, although triglyceride fat is also is a natural part of the body. Elevated levels of triglycerides in the blood are medical markers of excessive bad or undesirable fat. A measurement of triglycerides is included in a standard lipid profile.) In recent years, more and more has been written about correlations between consuming high fructose corn syrup and obesity. Also, there are some correlations between high fructose corn syrup and type II diabetes.

One's own doctor is the final authority, and her recommendations and guidelines should be closely followed. The dietary suggestions in Plan A and Plan B must not be used if they conflict with the recommendations of one's own doctor.

CHAPTER FIVE

THE PRINCETON STUDY

Representatives of the Corn Refiners Association and American soft drink companies have consistently argued that sucrose, corn syrup, and high fructose corn syrup are essentially the same. High fructose corn syrup, sucrose, and corn syrup are all commonly-used ingredients in processed foods and beverages. There are major similarities between all three substances. All three have high levels of calories. The calories of the three sweeteners are called "empty" because they lack nutrients. All three sweeteners are effective at sweetening, but HFCS is chemically different than sucrose and corn syrup. The manufacturing process of high fructose corn syrup produces a xenobiotic, foreign substance with broken chemical bonds.

The radical difference between old-time corn syrup and high fructose corn syrup is the chemical composition. Corn syrup is composed of glucose and fructose, as they were created in nature. (Fructose is generally metabolized in the liver. Glucose is used in every cell of the body.) High fructose corn syrup has glucose and fructose, also.

However, in addition, high fructose corn syrup has two unnatural parts.

High fructose corn syrup has unbound molecules, and it has a strange new "fructose" that was created, originally, by nature to be glucose. It appears that the bodies of those with fibromyalgia reject the synthetic fructose because chemically that portion of high fructose corn syrup is neither fructose nor glucose—at the level of metabolism. The synthetic "fructose" may have been close to natural fructose in the manufacturing plant. However, after the bodies' own enzymatic actions, the new "fructose" is transformed into an xenobiotic substance. The newly created "fructose" is a problem for metabolism. Those who argue that sucrose, corn syrup, and high fructose corn syrup are essentially the same are partially correct. Immediately after the manufacturing process, the three substances are almost the same. However, they are incorrect about their chemical nature of high fructose corn syrup once it is digested and is subjected to metabolism. Rodent and human bodies are adversely affected.

Several years ago, there were reports of an experiment with rats and high fructose corn syrup. The researchers fed rats high fructose corn syrup for a period of time. Eventually, the organs of the rats were significantly damaged. Researchers reported that some hearts of the rats burst after excessive use of high fructose corn syrup. Many of the male rats were no longer capable of reproduction because of damage to the testes. The female rats appeared to have been less harmed, but they could not reproduce. Examinations of blood content revealed a decline in copper levels. (Copper is an essential mineral that is needed for growth and cell repair.)

The critics claim that the study lacked sufficient controls, and numerous others substances (other than HFCS) might also cause damage if they were administered in excessive amounts. In addition, many argued that humans would not get a proportionately huge amount of high fructose corn syrup in typical daily diets, even over an extended period of time. To summarize the position of the critics, they argued that this rat study of high fructose corn syrup was flawed, and it would not be appropriate to compare or transfer the results to people. Critics claimed that there was a lack of compelling evidence supporting the view that HFCS is damaging to humans.

In 2010, researchers from the Department of Psychology at Princeton University and from the Princeton Neuroscience Institute designed and directed two well-controlled studies. These studies were supported by the U.S. Public Health Services. The first study was done for a shorter period of time, but it lead into the second study which has attracted a great deal of attention.

Male Sprague-Dawley rats were divided into two groups. One group of rats (the control group) was fed measured amounts of cane sugar water and rat chow. The experimental group was fed high fructose corn syrup and rat chow in equal proportions to the control group. Care was taken to administer the same portion sizes with the same caloric count to each group of rats. Although the reports read that the calorie counts were equal, at a later discussion, it was stated that if there was any difference in calorie count between the two groups, the HFCS group was the group that received slightly less calories.

In addition, the amount of high fructose corn syrup was reported to be proportional to the level a human would consume if he or she drank one sweetened carbonated beverage with other foods at a meal. The experiment lasted for more than six months. The rats were measured and monitored on three scales, periodically—weight gain, body fat, and triglyceride levels. Twenty-five to twenty-eight weeks later, the results were in.

The researchers reported that there were significant differences in the two rat groups on all three measurements. The HFCS rats had higher triglyceride levels (a condition called hyper-triglyceridemia in humans), had greater amounts of body fat (especially around the abdomen), and gained significantly more weight. It was reported that the average HFCS rat weighed nearly forty-eight percent more than the average sugar rat at the end of the experiment. Therefore, the HFCS rats consumed the same number of calories, or just slightly less, but they gained much more weight.

The scientific world and medical world have maintained that there are three, and only three, factors that affect weight gain and weight loss. The factors are 1) calories consumed 2) calories expended and 3) rate of metabolism. Assuming that these diet factors are as true for rats as they are for humans, then there are some remaining questions left over from the Princeton experiments. How did HFCS affect the rats in such a way that even though they were fed equal calories (or slightly less), they gained substantially more weight? The sugar rats stayed in their normal rat weight ranges.

Only two factors remain that could account for the different weight gain—activity level (energy expended) and rate of metabolism. It is possible that the high fructose corn syrup rats became less active, and the rats were slowed also by a stalled metabolism. The Princeton study gives compelling evidence that sugar and high fructose corn syrup act differently in the body—at least for rats.

A problem with using rats for studies of fibromyalgia is that the rats cannot talk and report their level of pain. Rats cannot communicate if they are dizzy or stiff. They won't complain about hesitating to climb a flight of stairs because of exhaustion. As limited as rats studies are, sometimes rat studies are one of the best experimental tools. Controlling rat environments is more practical and feasible than attempting to control the environment of humans. In addition, if harm comes to rats, it is considered less evil than harming humans or primates.

The HFCS Princeton rats may have lacked the energy needed for their usual level of activity. It is also possible that their overall metabolic processes were significantly slowed.

The Princeton study was not designed to provide insights into fibromyalgia. In fact, fibromyalgia has never been mentioned in conjunction with these experiments. However, because of common links, especially the link of high fructose corn syrup, the results are relevant to the study of fibromyalgia.

There are parallels between the results of rat studies and comparisons of medical reports of humans. Scientists have verified that triglyceride levels in humans are raised to higher levels following regular consumption of high fructose corn syrup.

There are several other medical issues that have negative correlations resulting from high fructose corn syrup use. Medical doctors and others believe that HFCS consumption is strongly linked with growing obesity rates in the U.S. and other countries. Some anecdotal reports of people suffering with fibromyalgia include statements regarding a slowed metabolism, as evidenced by shallow rates of respiration and chronic fatigue beginning several days after consuming high fructose corn syrup.

The implications of the Princeton study are profound and may be used as starting points for future research. Important remaining questions from the 2010 Princeton study are:

1.) Did the metabolism of the HFCS rats slow significantly?

2.) Did the HFCS rats exhibit significantly less activity?

3.) Were both the metabolic rates and the activity rates of the HFCS rats significantly different than the measurements of the sugar water rats?

Researchers at Duke University studied 427 adult patients who had been previously diagnosed with non-alcoholic fatty liver disease.

The report mentioned "fructose." Fructose is a natural sugar that occurs in many fruits and some vegetables. Therefore, it is possible that fruit juices and beverages were lumped together with high fructose corn syrup beverages.

Nineteen percent of the patients did not drink fructose-containing beverages. Fifty-two percent of participants had one to six fructose beverages each week. The remaining twenty-nine percent drank one or more beverages containing fructose every day. Statistical analysis and medical review of the three groups revealed that scarring in the liver occurs significantly more in those who regularly consume fructose beverages. The livers of those who did not drink fructose-containing beverages were the least scarred.

The overall ill effects of high fructose corn syrup on the health of consumers in the United States and throughout the world are becoming increasingly apparent to practicing physicians. Many doctors advise obese patients or patients with type II diabetes to avoid high fructose corn syrup. Some doctors are labeling symptoms resulting from HFCS consumption, "high fructose corn syrup sensitivity."

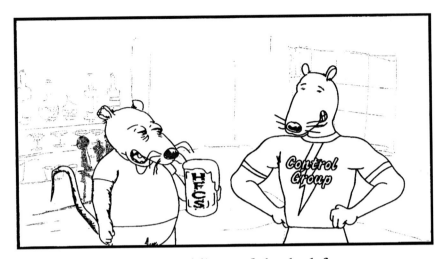

"Call me gullible! They said that high fructose
corn syrup is just like sugar!"

CHAPTER SIX

THE MANUFACTURE OF HIGH FRUCTOSE CORN SYRUP

Almost two hundred years ago, a process for creating corn syrup was developed, and this old-time corn syrup has remained a popular product since that time. Hydrolysis, a method of acid conversion, was used to convert corn starch to corn syrup. Corn syrup is a sweetening ingredient used in cooking and baking. Corn is plentiful in North America, and the process to convert corn starch to corn syrup is relatively simple. The basic chemical bonds of corn DNA are not changed during the hydrolysis process of old-time corn syrup.

Most reports indicate that high fructose corn syrup was invented in a laboratory in Japan in the 1960s. It was introduced to food manufacturers in the United States around 1970. A few companies began to manufacture and market high fructose corn syrup in 1976. Throughout several decades, HFCS has been used more and more frequently to replace cane and beet sugar in thousands of processed food products.

Like corn syrup, high fructose corn syrup begins as corn starch. Other similarities between corn syrup and high fructose corn syrup are their lack of nutrients, sweetening properties, high caloric content, and names. However, the complicated manufacturing process of high fructose corn syrup results in a denatured substance with DNA that is no longer shared with corn.

The manufacturing process converts a food into a semi-food. HFCS is an anomaly in the food world. It acts as food in the early stages of digestion, but it causes havoc at the cellular level for many people who have fibromyalgia.

The conversion of corn starch to high fructose corn syrup requires many steps. Two enzymes are utilized—alpha-anylase and glucoamylase. (Glucoamylase is an enzyme that is derived from a fungus.) The enzymes are added at different stages of production. Some have reported that a bacteria is also added to the mixture, although the name of the bacteria was not disclosed. Heating and cooling strengthen the enzymatic applications of the mixture. Near the end of the process a "fixative" is applied.

The manufacturing process reduces the level of glucose to less than half of the substance and increases the amount of fructose. The chemical bonds are broken in the manufacturing process and the left-over, synthetic irregular substance is referred to as "high sugar." It is reported that the substance with broken chemical bonds accounts for little more than three percent of the total HFCS mixture. Many refer to broken, free molecules as "free radicals." Free radicals are miniscule enough to slip through the pores of the intestinal membrane and reach the circulatory system. (Obviously, millions of food molecules pass through the intestinal membrane also. However, those food molecules have been prepared for further, natural metabolic use.) Currently, the exact chemical reactions of these free radicals on cells, other molecules, and neurotransmitters are not fully understood. It is believed that free radicals have the potential to travel all through the body, including the brain.

High fructose corn syrup is devoid of nutrients and is high in calories, but the most horrendous characteristic of this denatured substance is that, for millions of people, it confounds and stalls the metabolic processes. Its toxic properties temporarily affect the cells and central nervous system. There are no reports of deaths from high fructose corn syrup; however, the toxic, foreign component of the substance affects many in a way that is similar to that of a mild poison.

Some chemists have written of concerns regarding the purity of the enzymes used in the HFCS processing. They suspect that some contaminates may become a part of high fructose corn syrup. Some scientists who are focused on resolving issues of weight gain and obesity believe the unequal proportion (fructose to glucose) of high fructose corn syrup has a role in facilitating weight gain. They suspect that the high level of fructose in HFCS is converted into fat relatively quickly and easily. More steps are needed by the body for cane or beet sugar metabolism. Those additional chemical steps for the metabolism of cane and beet sugar are natural steps.

The unbound, free molecules of high fructose corn syrup appear to be a primary factor or a co-factor in the all-over pain, fatigue and stiffness of fibromyalgia. Free radicals can travel throughout the whole body and reach the central nervous system and the fascia.

Evidently, the final "fixative" application in the manufacturing process of HFCS is not powerful enough to withstand human metabolism. Explanations are needed on the following:

- the possible contamination of enzymes used in processing

- details on the chemical nature of the HFCS fixative

- implications of the disproportion of glucose and fructose

- the route and actions of free radicals in human metabolism

- synthetic fructose effects on the intestine, liver, and cells

CHAPTER SEVEN

METABOLISM AND XENOBIOTICS

Digestion is the process that begins with eating and chewing food into small substances. Enzymes and hydrochloric acid begin to work in the mouth to break food into smaller components. Part of metabolism involves the chemical processes that break the components into even smaller molecules in preparation for use by the cells. Enzymes work in the stomach, liver, and intestine for participation in these complicated chemical processes.

The pancreas (gland of the endocrine system) manufactures enzymes. Enzymes are proteins and chemicals that basically act as catalysts spurring on metabolism. The number of enzymes in the human body have been estimated to be more than seventy-five thousand. Some researchers have concluded that the number of enzymes is so great that even rough estimates are specious.

Enzymes influence the speed of metabolism. Although they interact with food molecules, they do not merge with or become a part of food molecules. In essence, they retain their own separate identities and usually work again at a later time with other food molecules (usually of the same food type). At some point, it appears that each enzyme loses its power and its ability to catalyze molecules.

One of the important roles of enzymes is to remove toxins from the body. Poisons decrease the production of enzymes. Therefore, a lower level of enzymes makes ridding the body of toxins more difficult. Some of the work of removing poisons and toxins from the body occurs in the small intestine.

Most understand that the intestine is a route of exit for body waste. In addition, the intestine has other important functions. The intestine significantly contributes to critical body and mind functioning. Serotonin is created in both the intestine and the brain. However, greater amounts of serotonin are created in the intestine. Serotonin is a neurotransmitter (hormone) that is linked with feelings of happiness. Conversely, the lack of serotonin may contribute to depression or catastrophic thinking.

The brain contains receptors for serotonin. Serotonin communicates with and effects brain activities. Therefore, efficient functioning of the intestine affects transmission in the central nervous system and, ultimately, the pituitary-hypothalamus-adrenal axis which controls major body functions. The pituitary-hypothalamus-adrenal axis of the brain affects regulation of the endocrine system, cycles of sleep, and motor functions. Another neurotransmitter that contributes to feelings of well-being and contentment is dopamine. Canadian researchers have found that during pain, the dopamine levels in those with fibromyalgia are significantly lower than the dopamine levels in those who do not have fibromyalgia. It is not clear whether the dopamine lessens prior to the pain or whether the pain contributes to the lower levels of dopamine.

Xenobiotics are foreign (strange) substances that contain unbound or toxic molecules. Molecules that contribute to efficient, healthy and natural metabolism are bound. (Typically, they are bound to protein molecules.) Unbound molecules are "free." The unbound molecules can enter the bloodstream, reach every part of the body, and damage soft tissue.

Reactions to xenobiotics are different from the body's reactions to food allergies. If the body is allergic to a food (good food examples are peanuts and shellfish), negative effects begin right after eating the food. There may be itching in the throat or ear canals and even the tongue and lips can swell. More violent reactions follow the earlier symptoms. In short, food allergies occur very quickly after ingesting the offensive substance—as quickly as seconds later.

Part of high fructose corn syrup and xenobiotics do no cause immediate reactions. They become disruptive and troublesome at later stages of metabolism.

Metabolism and life are inseparable. Metabolism begins at the beginning of life and continues until death. Metabolism is the process of providing nutrients and oxygen to aid in repair functions, cellular activity, gland functioning, etc. The activities of communication by the central nervous system, motor activities and thinking are all assisted with metabolism.

Complex chemical processes of metabolism work continuously. A depressed metabolism impacts neurotransmission and overall body functions.

High fructose corn syrup seems innocuous when eating and at the early stages of digestion. However, part of high fructose corn syrup (the synthetic part) is an anomaly to the metabolic process and is toxic to those with fibromyalgia. Most of the negative internal reactions to high fructose corn syrup are not felt on the first day of consumption. Reactions are rarely noticed during digestion of the large food molecules. The initial affects of a distressed metabolism usually become noticeable a few days after consumption of the substance.

The natural DNA in corn is transformed during the manufacturing process of high fructose corn syrup. The transformation from a natural product to high fructose corn syrup requires heating and cooling, back-blending, the application of enzymes during two or three stages of processing, and a chemical fixative. The result of a complicated manufacturing process is a substance that is synthetic and contains unbound molecules. Unbound molecules and synthetic fructose appear to play major roles in the pain, fatigue, and misery of fibromyalgia.

High fructose corn syrup, and other xenophobic substances, plays crucial roles in the distressing, widespread pain and chronic fatigue of fibromyalgia.

Chapter Eight

CAUSES OF FIBROMYALGIA

Fibromyalgia is caused by inorganic substances conflicting with or stalling the body's metabolism. Fibromyalgia is caused by man-made xenophobic molecules, quasi-foods, or both. Many of the symptoms of fibromyalgia occur at the molecular level of metabolism, during the time period that the molecules of the inorganic substances are circulating in the blood and affecting the organs and cells.

Inorganic substances include some man-made xenobiotics and foods that have been radically changed in manufacturing processes. Some manufactured foods are highly corrupt. The natural DNA of the original, biological food is changed; and the original chemical bonds are broken by the end of the manufacturing process.

The antagonistic inorganic molecules are specific for each person. He or she may react to only one or may react to several different food and beverage sources. Each person is genetically unique so his or her set of causes (or cause) may differ from those of others.

Xenobiotics

Natural xenobiotics (such as arsenic, hemlock, or poison from a puffer fish) potentially can stop metabolism completely and end life. Natural xenobiotics can result in severe toxic and fatal poisoning. However, natural xenobiotics are organic and are not typically associated with fibromyalgia symptoms.

Man-made xenobiotics are not organic. Many impede metabolism and cause dysfunction before expulsion from the body. Some man-made xenobiotics are linked with fibromyalgia symptoms. Man-made xenobiotics include chemicals such as malathion, chemical pesticides and insecticides, monosodium glutamate (MSG), and aspartame. Typically, only small amounts are consumed. (However, smallness does not mean an element or molecule is not extremely potent and toxic.) It is assumed that the body ultimately expels most of the toxic molecules through natural elimination processes.

High Fructose Corn Syrup

High fructose corn syrup contains some natural glucose and natural fructose. However, a portion of high fructose corn syrup is unnatural and inorganic. Considerable processing is done with heating and cooling, enzyme applications, back-blending and an application of a fixing agent. This inorganic portion of high fructose corn syrup causes problems for many people. Because the symptoms begin to be noticed two, three, or even four days after ingestion, many do not recognize the cause and effect relationships. The time lull between eating and feeling symptoms obscures the link. It is difficult to make the connection between an ingredient that was eaten two or three days ago and uncomfortable developing symptoms. Usually, most people do not recall the types of foods they ate days two or three days ago, let alone the ingredients of those processed foods.

Problems caused by high fructose corn syrup are disguised and hidden for several reasons. The cause and effect relationship is not usually recognized by the individual. The FDA labeled high fructose corn syrup as GRAS (meaning, generally recognized as safe.) In addition, many Americans have traditionally trusted manufacturers to be protective of them. Therefore, the cause of problems, that result from a synthetic and inorganic portion of high fructose corn syrup, has been disguised and hidden. Recent research has contributed to deeper understanding and will, in time; help illuminate this obscure, unfortunate connection.

Webster's Ninth New Collegiate Dictionary, published by Merriam-Webster in 1984, does not include either the word "high fructose corn syrup" or the word "fibromyalgia" because when words were collected and compiled for that edition of the dictionary, neither of the words were in use. High fructose corn syrup had been invented and had been manufactured for use in processed foods starting in the mid 1970s. However, at that time, high fructose corn syrup may have been seen as just a type of the long-used, plain corn syrup. Until the 1970s there were no reports of the collection of symptoms that is now called "fibromyalgia." Researchers claim the malady was first given its current name in the early 1980s. Therefore, both words were not included in Webster's 1983 dictionary. I believe that this "coincidence" of exclusion from dictionaries is more than just coincidence. Spaces are left in the following lists for your personal use.

Linked With Fibromyalgia

Inorganic substances in quasi-foods:

- High fructose corn syrup

- _____

Inorganic, man-made xenobiotics included in foods:

- Monosodium glutamate (MSG)

- Aspartame

- _____

Inorganic, man-made xenophobic residue, particles, or fumes:

- Harsh toxins used in oven cleaners

- Chemical pesticides and insecticides

- Substandard water

- _____

Not all of the above listed substances result in problems for each individual. Although some of the above substances may not cause specific pain or fatigue problems, none of them are considered healthy ingredients.

The above lists do not include all inorganic substances that cause fibromyalgia. Completion of the list will require further research, study, and statistical validation. Although the study is not yet complete, following the guidelines of this book should result in significant or nearly total relief from fibromyalgia symptoms for almost everyone.

CHAPTER NINE

FROM UPTON SINCLAIR TO XENOBIOTICS

At the beginning of the twentieth century, conditions in meat processing plants were harsh and unsafe for workers. Shoddy practices were regularly used in butchering and packaging meats. Product safety was given inadequate attention. In general, regulations, standards, and enforcement were deficient or lacking.

Upton Sinclair's novel, "The Jungle", shocked readers with its descriptions of fingers lost, human parts mixed into meat, filth on the shoes and clothing of workers, and the lack of regard for everyone's safety. After the book's distribution, a black and white film was made of the story. The book and the movie stirred the public's feelings of empathy for the workers, who were mostly immigrants from Europe. Many consumers were enraged when they realized that they had been eating unhygienic and, sometimes, contaminated meats and meat by-products.

Public opinion reached the representatives, Congress and the White House. "The Jungle" is credited with inspiring the 1906 Pure Food and Drug Act. President Theodore

Roosevelt signed the act which was referred to for some years, as the Wiley Act (last name of a researcher of that time period.)

The Pure Food and Drug Act is responsible for improving some worker safety conditions and enhancing food cleanliness and quality. In addition, all medicinal products are required to include the names of all ingredients on the product container.

After the Food and Drug Act was implemented into law, the U.S. Food and Drug Administration (FDA) was established. In 1938, the name of the first act was replaced with a new name, the Food, Drug, and Cosmetics Act. Over time, the guidance, testing, oversight, and approval responsibilities were expanded to include new areas and many new products, including tobacco and medical devices. In 2010, the Food Safety Modernization Act was implemented. Amendments and additional laws work together along with the original acts to form a comprehensive public health program.

The FDA has numerous divisions and branches and is responsible for multiple health and safety issues. The FDA staff has developed and published guidelines covering a multitude of areas, including imported fruit safety, "small entities," the amount of arsenic allowed in drinking water, and proper and explicit labeling on product labels. The quantity of materials produced by the administration is overwhelming, and the pages of the written guidelines number into the thousands. Prior to the marketing and distribution of new drugs, pharmaceutical companies must document and present their findings and test results to the FDA. The FDA has the legal power to reject or give approval to new products.

In recent decades, some pharmaceutical products received approval for marketing, were marketed, and then were "recalled" a couple of years later, or even several years later. Some deaths occurred and, in some instances, serious health problems developed because of early release or inadequate testing and review practices. Many years ago, thalidomide was prescribed for women who were burdened with nausea in pregnancy. Many of the babies born from these pregnancies presented with unformed limbs. Of course, thalidomide is no longer prescribed for pregnant women.

A drug that is a combination of an appetite suppressant and a hydrochloride, used by some to treat obesity, had a short period of popularity. Phen-fen acted quickly to speed up metabolism. It was quite effective in meeting its goal of weight reduction. However, medical reports of the side effects caused its recall and usage was discontinued. Regular usage resulted in a very serious side effect. Phen-fen damaged heart valves of many users.

A few partial foods that consist of a strange, synthetic part have been treated too leniently and have avoided testing and scrutiny—as if they were completely and wholly real foods. Synthetic substances, such as drugs, must be submitted to stricter review and standards than food. Trans fats and high fructose corn syrup are two substances that avoided testing and the review of an approval panel because they are partial foods. High fructose corn syrup was being used commercially before it received its GRAS (generally recognized as safe) status.

In the 1970s and 1980s, consumers purchased products such as cooking oil, peanut butter, margarine, salad dressings and baked goods that contained high levels of trans fats. Clinical reports of patient health problems and experiment results from animal studies combined to prove that trans fats directly relate to health risks, especially with the heart and arteries. Many consumers are now aware of the risks of consuming too much fat. Federal guidelines require that the percent of trans fat or amount of trans fat be listed on ingredient labels.

In 1983, high fructose corn syrup was given GRAS status by the FDA. There are a few reports that suggest that high fructose corn syrup was given leniency partially because of a cozy relationship between the Corn Refiners Association and managers of the FDA.

It is possible that some in the FDA considered high fructose corn syrup a natural food—perhaps a close cousin of plain corn syrup. It isn't known whether an FDA panel, at the time of product review, was given information on the manufacturing process of high fructose corn syrup. The production and use of high fructose corn syrup continued to grow as more and more manufacturers chose to add it into their existing food products.

The FDA is well-organized and respected as an institution. Its work is essential to consumer safety. Some claim that the FDA is understaffed considering the very high volume of work and complexity of the review processes. Approximately a thousand new chemicals are created each year. It is estimated that there are more than seventy thousand chemicals used commercially in the United States.

The panels, scientists, and support staff of the FDA are pressured to work quickly to ultimately hasten the approval of products. Pharmaceutical companies and corporations representing the American agri-business community push to get their products approved to meet the goals of gaining new revenue sources.

Some of these corporations are powerful and considered icons to business and commercial industries. Some insiders of the FDA admit there are a few cases in which prudence was compromised in exchange for expedience and amicable relationships between FDA reviewers and corn industry representatives.

Many believe that the FDA has made a few mistakes by giving GRAS status to both high fructose corn syrup and monosodium glutamate and by giving FDA approval to aspartame. Many hope those decisions will be rescinded. The three food additives that are of the greatest concern for people with fibromyalgia are high fructose corn syrup, monosodium glutamate, and aspartame.

High Fructose Corn Syrup

High fructose corn syrup was added to many products beginning in the mid 1970s. Every year more and more manufacturers found reasons to use it. High fructose corn syrup is relatively inexpensive; it acts as a preservative; it is very sweet; it acts as a humectants (retains moisture); it is stable at different temperatures; it has an attractive consistency for syrups, ice cream, salad dressings and other products; and it is easy to mix in with other products. A few years later, high fructose corn syrup was added to crackers, cereals, bagels, canned soup, cold cereals, yogurt, bread, ketchup, spaghetti sauce, cookies, and numerous other products. In the 1980s and 1990s the production and use of high fructose corn syrup grew exponentially.

For many years, most people accepted high fructose corn syrup as a junk food additive, but a relatively harmless food additive. Most employees of the FDA were not aware of the detrimental effects of high fructose corn syrup. High fructose corn syrup was in use commercially for almost eight years before the FDA gave it GRAS status.

Arguments were presented years ago, and continue currently, regarding superficial observations of similarities between the composition of high fructose corn syrup and the tried-and-true, much-used original corn syrup. Although both have calories and are derivatives of corn, they can cause very different reactions for metabolic functions. Fructose and glucose (major components of high fructose corn syrup) are metabolized differently. Fructose metabolism is generally limited to the liver. Glucose is required for energy production all over the body and is used continuously by every cell throughout the body. The glaring remaining question on metabolism of high fructose corn syrup is how is the synthetic portion of high fructose corn syrup treated at the metabolic level.

The guidelines of the FDA regarding the use of the term "organic" bar manufacturers of high fructose corn syrup from describing their products as "organic.". Currently, some activists are requesting that the FDA also disallow the term "natural" on products containing HFCS.

The growing evidence of the irregular and negative effects of high fructose corn syrup on metabolism is getting more attention. The results of the Princeton study and the correlations between incidences of obesity and consumption of high fructose corn syrup have re-opened the debate on the GRAS status.

Many have reported consistent negative experiences with fibromyalgia after consuming high fructose corn syrup. The efforts of biochemists and endocrinologists are needed to document the metabolic interactions and the route of free molecules of high fructose corn syrup through the bloodstream and central nervous system. High fructose corn syrup has not yet been labeled an xenobiotic. It is strange mixture that is certainly foreign to the bodies of many, and appears to be a neurotoxin for those with fibromyalgia.

Monosodium Glutamate (MSG)

Monosodium glutamate (MSG) is a manufactured food additive that is an excitotoxin. As the name "excitotoxin" implies, it enhances the taste of food by exciting the nerves of the body beginning in the mouth. Monosodium glutamate is a food additive, but it does not contain anything flavorful. Rather MSG temporarily changes taste receptors. In addition to affecting taste buds, it also damages internal cells.

Like high fructose corn syrup, monosodium glutamate was given GRAS status by the FDA many years ago. The "Nutrition and healthy eating" section of the Mayo Clinic website states that even though it is generally recognized as safe, controversy over its nature has continued for some time (author's re-wording). Many symptoms are listed as reactions under the title "MSG Symptom Complex." Those symptoms include headaches, nausea, chest pain, heart palpitations, sweating, and weakness. Some reports say that more than eighty percent of adults experience some MSG sensitivity, such as diarrhea, headaches, and lightheadedness.

The argument that MSG in food is in such tiny amounts that MSG can do very little harm seems rather weak. One might eat several food products, in the same time period, that contain MSG, and MSG may have a cumulative effect. Consumer groups have requested that the FDA rescind the GRAS status for MSG. Excitotoxins, in general, have been linked to some serious conditions, including Parkinson's disease and Alzheimer's. The manufacturers argue that no substantive proof of the negative effects of MSG has been presented. Once a substance is frequently used by most in the population, it becomes very difficult to study its effects. Scientific experimentation and research require planning and manipulation so that only one variable is the variable responsible for the outcome, ideally.

Many scientists strongly believe that over time monosodium glutamate is very likely to directly harm or contribute to tissue harm of humans. Some are convinced, from animal study results, that severe permanent change will occur in the central nervous system and brain when used over a long period of time.

There are some scientists who believe that MSG and other excitotoxins may be relatively benign when used in small quantities. That idea begs the following question. What amounts and over how long a period of time does MSG become deleterious? In other words, how many years of use are likely to result in Parkinson's?

The plethora of products, multiple names of substances containing MSG, and the frequent use by processed food manufacturers and restaurants, make avoiding all MSG nearly impossible. The following names are some of the typical food additives that contain significant amounts of MSG: yeast extract, sodium caseinate, gelatin, textured protein, hydrolyzed protein, glutanic acid, and monopotassium glutanate.

Aspartame

Aspartame is an excitotoxin that is used as a sweetener. It sweetens food and beverages without adding any calories. Aspartame was accidentally discovered in 1965 by a pharmaceutical company. A patent was obtained in 1970. Many argued against its production and distribution for human use. Aspartame was not given GRAS status; however, the FDA approved aspartame for marketing in 1974—against the objections of many.

In numerous animal studies, aspartame proved to induce brain tumors and tumors in other organs. Most who reviewed the rat studies deemed the methodology and reports to be valid and reliable. Some of the FDA's own scientists argued against approving aspartame. Several FDA scientists who took a more lenient view or cavalier attitude toward product approval and release were later suspected of violations of conflict of interest policies.

Aspartame is marketed and distributed on a world-wide basis. The profits are so phenomenally large, it is difficult to find an adjective that truly describes the degree of greatness of the financial profits. In essence, the pharmaceutical companies who manufacture aspartame will certainly hire and engage the most effective scientists and attorneys they can find in order to continue the production, distribution, and sales.

An Italian study linked aspartame to lymphoma, especially in the brain, and leukemia. The researchers fed each animal aspartame throughout its whole life. After each animal's natural death, the body was dissected for study of internal abnormalities. Lymphoma and leukemia were seen in the subject rats.

Some studies point to aspartame as a carcinogen or as a co-carcinogen when interacting with other agents. Research is on-going and so are the debates.

A powerful preventive measure one can make for his or her health, with or without the problem of fibromyalgia, is to reject as many products as possible that contain either high fructose corn syrup, MSG, or aspartame.

Excitotoxins

Xenobiotics are substances that are foreign to the body. These substances or molecules are strange and irregular, and they are not similar to the natural biological and chemical qualities of food, water, and air. Research on xenobiotics is a relatively new branch of science. Excitotoxins are a particular type of xenobiotics that are in food and beverages. Xenobiotics is a broader term that covers food, particulates in air, and pesticide residue.

MSG and aspartame are well-known neurotoxins and excitotoxins, and they remain in the forefront of discussions and debate for scientists and consumers.

Dr. Russell Blaylock has been writing and teaching about the dangers of excitotoxins since the 1990s. Online research of his background reveals his esteemed status in the scientific community. Dr. Blaylock is a practicing medical doctor with years of medical experience. In addition, he is a successful lecturer, professor, and author. His medical specialty is neurosurgery. Dr. Blaylock is a recipient of an award for "Integrity in Science" by the Westin Price Foundation. The focus of some of Dr. Blaylock's work is environmental factors and human health. His book, "Excitotoxins: The Taste That Kills" has received much acclaim. Currently, Dr. Blaylock serves on the editorial staff of the "Journal of the American Nutracentrical Association" and on the editorial staff of the "Journal of American Physicians and Surgeons."

Dr. Blaylock and others believe that cancer growth and cancer metastasis are rapidly increased by the use of excitotoxins. Dr. Blaylock and other scientists believe that excitotoxins promote the development of neurological disorders such as migraines, seizures, and infections. There may also be links with some endocrine disorders.

Many have great concerns over the role of excitotoxins in the development of Parkinson's, ALS, Huntington's disease, and Alzheimer's. Many of these neurological diseases share common factors of irregularities in central nervous system processing and of slow development over time. Symptoms that begin later in life sometimes indicate gradual accumulation of toxins. In contrast, the order of fibromyalgia symptoms and the cyclical or intermittent nature of fibromyalgia seem to indicate the body's rejection of toxins at the metabolic level. Rejection, rather than accumulation, could be one positive attribute of fibromyalgia.

Chapter Ten

Fascia, Pain, and the Central Nervous System

Fascia is a type of connective tissue that consists of collagen, elastin, nerve endings and fibroblasts. It is part of connective tissue that surrounds muscles, organs, intestine, bones and muscle. It runs continuously throughout the body like an envelope for everything under the skin. Much of the fascia lies just beneath the skin. Some fascia surrounds intestine and organs deep within the body. The nervous system and circulatory system converge in the fascia. The fascia helps to hold the body together, sustain the physique, and support and separate organs and muscles. Its appearance is a whitish, semi-opaque membrane. A good example of fascia is the thin, stretchy membrane between the skin and the meat of a raw chicken breast.

Prior to 2005, there were no illustrations of fascia in anatomy or biology textbooks. Because little was known about the functions of the fascia before the 21st century, scientists and medical personnel gave it little attention.

Massage therapists and a few others were the first to understand the fascia's important role in pain, relaxation, body comfort, posture and general well-being. In the last decade, the scientific community has given more attention to the roles of fascia. In 2007, researchers gathered at a conference for review and discussions at the first International Fascia Research Congress. Research on fascia is on-going.

Injuries, trauma, immobility, poor posture, and periods of fibromyalgia effect the fascia. Although fascia appears thin, it is strong and can be very forceful. Fibromyalgia problems of the fascia are significant and certainly degrade the quality of life. The feeling of being tight, constricted, and constrained through the back, neck, and shoulders is almost miserable.

Fascia that is in optimal condition is very elastic and moves easily over the musculoskeletal system. It protects internal organs; helps support the head, muscles and bones; and stretches and contracts to facilitate movement and physical activity.

The connective tissue of the lumbar (torso) of the body consists of cells that have a higher (or denser) concentration of fibroblasts than the connective tissue on the arms and legs. The denser concentration of fibroblasts in the back and neck may account for the location of pain and unrelenting stiffness for those suffering with fibromyalgia. Complaints of pain or stiffness in the lower legs or lower arms are rare. Impaired fascia becomes tighter and more immobile in the neck, upper back, shoulders and mid and lower back. There is less tightness and restriction in parts of the body that are the greatest distance from the central nervous system. The spinal cord, running up the back and through the neck, and the brain are the two subparts of the central nervous system.

The great discomfort and stiffness from fibromyalgia can be eased with the help of a masseuse or one who practices acupressure. Some find that all-over relief from tightness and compression does not happen until the bout of fibromyalgia is near completion. However, massage of the fascia provides some comfort. Research has not yet provided definitive answers on what happens in the body that results in less flexibility and stretchiness.

To create high fructose corn syrup the chemical bonds are broken and rearranged (denatured). Left over from this manufacturing process are unbound, free molecules. Noxious substances or an xenobiotic portion of the high fructose corn syrup are not metabolized as normal food. Instead, it appears that the body treats xenobiotic molecules as poison at a later stage of metabolism.

I am suggesting that the stiffness in the fascia either results from foreign enzymes or from unbound particles (from broken chemical bonds) adhering to fibroblasts or elastin causing a diminished capacity for stretchiness. To create high fructose corn syrup the chemical bonds are broken and rearranged. Left over from this manufacturing process are unbound molecules. When the chemical bonds of the glucose from corn syrup are broken and rearranged, the basic DNA of the corn syrup is changed. A complicated process is needed to change natural glucose into "high fructose". I suspect the body's metabolism is stalled by a substance that meets neither the standards of fructose nor glucose.

The denatured element of HFCS consists of small molecules that easily pass through membrane into the bloodstream. The capillaries of the blood supply run in a network throughout the fascia. The receptors of the nervous system and the blood stream, carrying foreign, denatured molecules, converge in the fascia.

The fascia and almost all soft tissue of the body contain pain receptors. (The brain and parts of the intestine do not contain pain receptors.) The ligaments, tendons, and muscles contain millions of pain receptors. Pain receptors connect with the central nervous system. Whether pain originates on the surface of the body or from inside the body, neurotransmitters connect with the central nervous system and signal pain.

The thalamus is an area of the brain that is made up of neurons (nerve cells). The thalamus, as part of the central nervous system, plays a part in neural coordination and pain processing. There is evidence of lower levels of activity in the thalamus of those diagnosed with fibromyalgia. In addition, pain inhibitory pathways and pain facilitatory pathways in the central nervous system of those with fibromyalgia behave irregularly during periods of pain. Serotonin levels and dopamine levels appear to be depressed when metabolism is burdened with toxins. The differences in the activity of the central nervous system may account for the reports of heightened sensitivity to pain by fibromyalgia sufferers. In addition, the "happy" hormones, serotonin and dopamine, are in short supply.

To summarize, the pain and achiness of those with fibromyalgia result, in part, from contracted fascia restricting and applying pressure to the muscles, tendons, ligaments and organs. Abnormal processing in the pathways of the central nervous system may exacerbate the degree of pain. Lower levels of dopamine and serotonin also detract from feelings of well-being.

Fibromyalgia pain is "real," but those with fibromyalgia have pathways in the central nervous system that work slowly (inhibition) to relay the message to the brain that the cause of the pain is subsiding. Compared with the healthy population, those with fibromyalgia are described as having greater sensitivity to pain ("overactive nerves").

CHAPTER ELEVEN

FATIGUE AND ENERGY

Fatigue sometimes creates a severe struggle for most who suffer from fibromyalgia. Many complain that even after hours of sleep, they still feel tired or even exhausted. During their worst periods, some sleep for a day or more and wake up every so often only to return to sleep after an hour or two of consciousness. Some suffering with fibromyalgia report that climbing a flight of stairs is exhausting and laborious.

Neither explanations of physical exhaustion nor explanations of emotional exhaustion account for the fibromyalgia fatigue. The fatigue is unrelated to strenuous exercise. Fibromyalgia fatigue results from a confounded metabolism and insufficient energy production in cells. (Unlike glucose's essential part in energy production, fructose has a limited part in energy production.)

The mitochondria (the "powerhouse" of the cells) produce energy. To produce the energy, the mitochondria need a constant supply of oxygen and glucose. Most fructose is metabolized in the cells of the liver. Glucose is metabolized in cells in all tissues and organs of the body. Glucose has a life-sustaining role. The relationship of free radicals, or unbound molecules, to energy production is not currently understood.

High fructose corn syrup (with a disproportionate amount of fructose) may overtax the liver. The mitochondria of the cells may not be able to use abnormal glucose that has been changed into something like synthetic fructose. The foreign substance may be close to a natural fructose in superficial ways, but it has a completely different chemical formula. Many argue that high fructose corn syrup is without a chemical formula. The synthetic "fructose" is sweet and easy to digest for most people. However, synthetic fructose is not the same to metabolism. Natural fructose and glucose have identified chemical formulae. The body's own enzymes may play a part in partial reversal of the manufacturing process. The part of high fructose corn syrup that is the new synthetic "fructose" is neither fructose nor glucose. It is a synthetic substance hanging in between the two, at the molecular level of the body.

Toxins in the body also decrease cellular function. Arsenic (found in some pesticides, insecticides and water supplies) disturbs glucose metabolism. Xenobiotics also disturb metabolism. Slowed and inefficient metabolism may contribute to the overall feeling of fatigue. A diminished supply of oxygen certainly contributes to fatigue. As discussed previously, the cells may produce less energy because of an inadequate amount of glucose or an unusable form of glucose (synthetic "fructose").

Chapter Twelve

UNDER THE RADAR

Radar is a system or device that spots an object and analyzes certain characteristics by the use of high frequency radio waves.

During World War II, radar devices were used as part of a defensive strategy to detect enemy planes in the sky. We can assume that the current usage of the expression "under the radar" is taken from that time when planes flying at lower altitudes were missed by radar. Therefore, they were under the radar.

The unbound molecules of the synthetic part of high fructose corn syrup have remained under the radar of many scientists, nutritionists, consumers, and people battling fibromyalgia for quite a long time. There are many obvious reasons for the hidden nature of high fructose corn syrup. Two very simples reasons are that high fructose corn syrup has disguised itself as a food, and that the culprit is too small to see with the naked eye. It is believed that when high fructose corn syrup was first manufactured, it inherited the reputation of old-time corn syrup. Simple corn syrup is chemically close to sugar.

Plain, old-time corn syrup has been a part of the American diet for more than a hundred years. Although it is deficient in nutrients, it is sweet and contains calories. Old-time corn syrup does not affect metabolism process in negative ways. Corn syrup has been widely accepted as innocuous for decades. Its reputation for being harmless and innocent has been so powerful that mothers and nurses have sometimes added corn syrup to the formula in baby bottles to be fed to their infants. The positive regard for the old-time corn syrup transferred to high fructose corn syrup and stuck with it for several years.

Because of the similarity of their names, it is easy to assume that corn syrup and high fructose corn syrup are almost the same or only mildly different. We now know the molecules of the two substances take very different paths at the molecular level of metabolism. Their essential DNA differs from one another. Corn syrup is chemically stable, and has retained the basic corn DNA. High fructose corn syrup contains free, unbound molecules, frequently referred to as "free radicals."

A visual sketch of a whole molecule of high fructose corn syrup shows a large part of the molecule as glucose (organic) and another large part of the molecule as fructose (organic) and sandwiched between the two large parts is a very small part labeled high fructose corn syrup. The very small part is less than four percent of the molecule so it is almost unnoticeable, nearly hidden. (This is a weak reason to explain being under the radar. It is basically a symbolic metaphor for the hidden issue.)

High fructose corn syrup is considered a food or a food additive. Typically, food is thought of as natural. Some of high fructose corn syrup—the high fructose part—is not healthy, not natural, and not organic.

The public relations and marketing representatives of the corn growers associations may prefer that the general public not hear any negative reports about their product and not be made aware of the complicated process required for high fructose corn syrup production. Certainly, industries that manufacture high fructose corn syrup hope to maintain a positive image. An untainted reputation can add to greater sales numbers for their product. In turn, sales will directly influence profit. High fructose corn syrup is relatively inexpensive to manufacture. The sale of HFCS ensures millions of dollars of profit every year. Protection and enhancement of the profits seem to outweigh the value of any other issue for marketing and public relations personnel. (When and if there is nearly total disregard for the issues of health and general welfare, the organization then loses both credibility and its moral compass.)

Another hidden part of high fructose corn syrup is its chemical formula. When asked for a formula, the answer becomes the standard formula for glucose or the standard formula for fructose. (Both glucose and fructose have identical chemical formulas.) Some have said that there is no formula for the "high fructose" part.

As discussed earlier, those suffering with fibromyalgia generally are not aware of the link between what they eat and drink and fibromyalgia symptoms. There is a long delay (two to four days, at least) between eating a small box of poor quality jelly beans or eating a plastic wrapped prepared muffin (containing HFCS) and all-over pain, fatigue and a slightly diminished state of consciousness. The long delay usually completely hides the cause and effect relationship.

Many assume that most food products are basically safe. It does not occur to many that a beverage or product consumed three days earlier is now being treated as a toxin at the molecular level of metabolism. Both the long delay between cause and effect and the positive regard many hold for food products overall, contribute to masking the real source of problems. On days three, four and five after ingestion, numerous fibromyalgia sufferers are perplexed and truly at lost for explanations. They ask silently to themselves, "What has happened?" or "What have I done wrong?"

Seeing the connections between high fructose corn syrup and fibromyalgia has presented a formidable challenge. All forms of communication will help in increasing awareness and understanding. One goal of this book is to help people understand the long delay between substance and symptoms. There is a very long delay between consumption and symptoms for the synthetic, manufactured substance, high fructose corn syrup.

CHAPTER THIRTEEN

FIBROMYALGIA, SCIENCE, AND RESEARCH

The research tools used for the materials of this book include observation, comparisons of anecdotal reports, and review and analysis of scientific experiments. All diseases, conditions, and medical problems have one or more causes. Fibromyalgia may have several different causes.

Medical science is sometimes explained as a field that is partially an art. The practice of medicine is related to art because it requires some imagination and creativity on the part of the physician. There are many variables related to symptoms and treatments. In addition, each body is unique.

Much of the medical world is supported by tests and observations of physical signs that reflect underlying internal dynamics. Doctors often rely on inference. They use experience, knowledge, and reasoning to arrive at very probable conclusions.

You may recall participating in the litmus paper test in school. You were not able to see what substance was an alkali and which was an acid. Once you dipped the paper into the liquid or applied the liquid to the paper, the paper changed to either a pink/red color or to a blue color. Therefore, by observing the new color of the paper, you were able to infer which substance was an acid and which was an alkaline liquid. Inference from test results is an important diagnostic tool.

The researchers and professors involved in the Princeton study of rats and high fructose corn syrup (Chapter Five) were not able to observe the molecules of high fructose corn syrup interacting with hormones, enzymes, and cellular activity. They inferred the interactions based on the average body weight of the rats at the end of the experiments and the significant increase in abdominal fat of each rat in the experimental group.

Currently, the causes of fibromyalgia must be identified through the process of reasoning and inference. The cause(s) of fibromyalgia are elusive; meaning proof of the most likely causes may not meet all scientific criteria for scientific proof. There are several formidable reasons why proof of fibromyalgia causes is difficult to obtain. Pinpointing exact causes supported by valid and reliable results requires controlled experiments and replication of successful experiments by others. (Replication is needed to ensure a degree of objectivity and counter human tendencies toward subjectivity.)

It is unethical to experiment with human beings if a treatment or substance has the potential to do great harm or long-term damage. In the case of fibromyalgia, the suspected toxins are in foods and beverages that are consumed daily by millions of Americans. The three most likely causal suspects of fibromyalgia are high fructose corn syrup, monosodium glutamate (MSG), and aspartame. They have been infused into carbonated beverages, fruit drinks, numerous types and varieties of processed foods, and a few food seasonings.

To use humans for a scientific study of high fructose corn syrup would require that dozens of people (subjects) be sequestered away from society and their everyday lives for several weeks. The following is a hypothetical experiment whose design involves controls, numerous volunteers who have fibromyalgia, careful oversight, dieticians, measurement, precise record keeping and very agreeable and cooperative volunteers. In addition to experimental requirements, the subjects need beds, toilets, paper products, soap, water, furniture, etc. The volunteers would have to arrange in advance for people to take over the necessary duties and obligations of their daily lives, because no one would be allowed to leave the facility for the duration of the experiment. The food, in this case, would be controlled by the researchers running the experiment and the hired dieticians.

Three equal groups of 25 subjects each would be a decent start for the experiment. The volunteers would be over the age of twenty one and would have been diagnosed with fibromyalgia at least one year earlier. All meals would be pre-planned and food carefully measured. The foods, meals, snacks, and beverages would be measured for uniformity in portion sizes. If all females volunteered as subjects, it would be easier to distribute the same size portions (because the need of males for more calories would not have to be dealt with). The only difference in the foods would be some would have foods that were sweetened only with sugar, honey or maple syrup (Group I). Group I would have no high fructose corn syrup in any food or beverage. The subjects in Group II would have a combination of some foods with high fructose corn syrup and other foods sweetened with sugar or honey. The amount of high fructose corn syrup in Group II would be small. Group III would have everything that needed to be sweetened, sweetened with high fructose corn syrup. Barbeque sauces, ketchup, salad dressings, muffins, rolls, bread, coffee creamers, pancake syrup, carbonated beverages, bottled lemonade, and cold cereals. (It is very easy to find plenty of foods with HFCS.) This experiment would ideally continue for six weeks.

It would be important that no subject be told of the exact nature of the experiment. The subjects would be given simple explanations of just "research for fibromyalgia." Also, no subject would know that there were three different food groups. Therefore, she would not know which group she was in because she would not realize the groups were being fed food that looked alike, but contain different ingredients. All the food would look like each comparable food for each group, and the foods would be very, very similar in taste. Portion size would be equal, and the subjects would be asked to eat everything. (If we keep the portions sizes at a moderate level, most will be hungry enough to enthusiastically eat all of their meals.)

On the first day, after everyone unpacks and gets settled into their very nice rooms. (Remember this is just hypothetical so they we might as well give them really plush accommodations.) Our subjects would be asked to sign contracts agreeing not to discuss their pain or discomfort with any other subjects until after their six week stay. Ideally, no one will become so sick during the experiment that she could not eat one of the meals. Hopefully, no one will have to leave and go home to attend to emergency situations with her child or pet. And, of course, we hope no one breaks the contract and discusses their level of pain or misery.

A well-accepted Visual Acuity Scale (VAS) would be used to measure pain, maybe at five day intervals. Subjects will be interviewed and report their levels of pain on the zero to ten pain scale. Measurements the first week would not be of too much value because everyone's body could have some food molecules from foods they had eaten prior to the experiment. So, lets take measurements and document pain levels at days 8, 13, 18, 23, 28, 33, and 38. The last four measurement days would be the most valuable for our experiment. After we gather all our data, lets thank everyone and let them go home. We can send them the results of the experiment a little later.

Our goal is to determine if HFCS consumption causes pain to our subjects. To analyze our data, we take the average (mean) score of each of the three groups on the VAS for day 23. A statistical formula is applied to each of the three groups to determine if there is enough of a difference between each average score of each group and average scores of each other groups to prove that high fructose corn syrup is related to their pain, lack of pain, or rather lesser feelings of pain. We apply the same statistical test for the day 28 data and again for day 33 and then again for day 38. A statistical test such as a "T" test yields data that reflects a measured difference in the means of the groups. If the results are significantly different, then there is more than a ninety-five percent chance that the difference in group means (averages) is the result of our experimental substance (in this case HFCS). There is less than a five percent chance that the result occurred because of chance.

This sounds like a lot of fun, but realistically it is a little impractical and totally hypothetical. The above experiment will probably not be conducted because of practical and economic issues.

Millions of dollars are spent for research and development of treatments of SYMPTOMS because of the possibility of great financial gain from never-ending treatments for never-ending symptoms. Pharmaceutical companies and the Corn Refiners Association cannot be counted on to give time or money to research intended to pinpoint exact causes of fibromyalgia.

If exclusion of certain food products is proven to be the cure, then no one would need pharmaceutical remedies and most would avoid high fructose corn syrup.

By now, I believe you understand the challenge to those studying fibromyalgia. Major challenges include expense, practicality and gathering enough willing participants with flexible lifestyles, and understanding employers and family members. In addition, symptoms of fibromyalgia cannot be observed by doctors or researchers. No chemical markers of internal body processes for fibromyalgia have been found, to date. (Therefore, measurement is limited.) Years ago, some believed that a substance "P" in the body was a chemical marker of pain in those with fibromyalgia. Because that discussion has not been included in current research materials, I assume the study of substance "P" has been discontinued because of unimpressive results. Measurement and documentation are critical components of science.

The goal of a scientific study is to have the substance in question be the one and only difference between two (or more) groups. All the other variables between the groups should be the same.

Here is a maxim from statistics, "correlation is not causality". Often you will hear of results with an announcement that this substance and that condition are correlated or linked. That means there may be a connection, but there is no real evidence or proof that one causes the other. It could be a statement that follows some casual observations or sums up a very weak experiment with inadequate controls of some of the variables. Correlations are not proof.

My professor stated, "People with big feet score higher on math tests than do people with small feet." He explained that it a true statement if you take into account all people of all ages. Children of ages four to eleven have much smaller feet than adults. Therefore, although the foot statement is true, it is only a correlation and does not indicate a cause and effect relationship between foot size and math test performance. The better math scores of adults are more likely related to maturation, education, and practice with arithmetic. Correlation here is definitely not causality.

You may recall the long struggle between the FDA and tobacco companies over the safety of cigarette smoking. The tobacco industry hired highly skilled lawyers and scientists to try to win their case. They argued that there was not enough scientific proof to fully prove that cigarette smoking causes lung cancer. To counter their arguments, many types of data were used, such as anecdotal reports, correlations, and results of animal studies (application of nicotine to the skin of rodents.) Although the tobacco industry was correct about the lack of genuine scientific proof with experiments on people, combining all the data from a variety of sources was convincing and compelling. The tobacco industry lost the case, in spite of the lack of the most stringent standards of scientific proof.

At times, corporations and agri-business fight to suppress information if the information can potentially reduce their profits. Some demand that critics prove that their products are harmful, even though the industry representatives know that no one proved that the products were safe before marketing them in the first place. That is the case for monosodium glutamate, aspartame, and high fructose corn syrup. All three are recognized as unhealthy by most in the scientific community.

When experiments with humans are impractical, unfeasible, or unethical, animals are used for experimentation. At times, monkeys are used. Generally it is more practical to use rodents such as rats or mice. Strict controls can be put in place for experiments with rats. It is fairly easy to observe them or remove them for measurements while they are contained in metal or glass cages. The results are transferred or extrapolated to similar conditions of people. Critics can charge that it might not be the same with humans. The internal system of people may be vastly different from the metabolic processes of rats, one might claim. There are great similarities, as well, in animal systems and people systems. Apes, of course, are biologically closest to humans.

Unfortunately, rats and monkeys usually are unable to rate their level of pain and report their pain experience to a clinician. Reports of pain are needed when studying fibromyalgia.

There is no easy way around all the roadblocks for fibromyalgia study. The researchers at Princeton University have taken the body of science on high fructose corn syrup a big step forward by their 2010 experiments. I believe results of the studies were first reported in a campus newspaper and later distributed to other forms of media. Their research proves, for many, that high fructose corn syrup affects the body very differently than sucrose. Although the calorie count given to each group of rats was the same, the rats consuming HFCS ended up weighing approximately forty-eight percent more than the sucrose fed rats. In addition, the weight gain was very noticeable as fat around the middle of the rats' torsos. The sucrose rats, with the same amount of calories, stayed within a normal weight range, and they were not obese.

Although the Princeton study was not focused on fibromyalgia, it does validate the hypothesis that high fructose corn syrup affects metabolism differently than sucrose—at least for rats.

Chapter Fourteen

INVISIBLE TO THE NAKED EYE

We cannot see the critical components of the metabolic processes in our bodies. The cells, enzymes, and neurotransmitters (hormones) are all too small to see with the naked eye. We cannot see the mitochondria and the ATP producing energy in cells. Similarly, we cannot see either synapses of nerves or fibroblasts in the fascia.

Since all activities, breathing, thinking, speaking, etc., are supported and fueled by metabolism, observing a live person or animal is observing the results of metabolism. We can see, hear, and feel the results of metabolism; but we cannot see the basic chemical processes of internal metabolism.

Physicians sometimes use pulse rates and equipment that measures the level of oxygen in the blood to assess the quality of metabolism. Without advanced education, the lay person is not equipped to study metabolism. He or she lacks the resources, tools and support to study issues such as enzymatic reactions and chemical catalysts, the paths and connections of neurotransmitters through the spinal cord and into the brain, cellular activities, serotonin and dopamine levels, and chemical activities which slow or speed rates of communication between all part of the body.

The primary problems of fibromyalgia—stiffness, all-over pain, chronic fatigue, and mild depression or catastrophic thinking—are also invisible. The levels of intensity of these problems must be revealed by those who are suffering. Of course, the reports may be somewhat subjective because the subjects are doing the reporting. Measures of fibromyalgia symptoms fall short of scientific accuracy.

The elements of high fructose corn syrup that are irregular and contribute to problems in metabolic processes are also too small to see. We cannot see the unbound molecules (free radicals) reacting on cells throughout the body, or the glucose being metabolized in cells in the muscles, or fructose being metabolized in the liver.

There are online and written documents on the harmful effects of aspartame and monosodium glutamate on cells in the body. Some results of the internal damage can be observed, such as breathing difficulties, swelling of the lips or tongue, diarrhea, or dizziness. However, the affected metabolic processes underlying the observable, external reactions, cannot be seen by casual observers.

The Princeton study on the effect of high fructose corn syrup on rats used measurement tools to compare the average weight of each group of rats with the average weight of the other rat group. In addition, researchers were able to measure the circulating triglyceride levels in the blood of the rats. However, few have the tools to observe the increasing or decreasing energy production in the cells. If the rats were experiencing any pain, the researchers would not be able to observe that process or measure the amount of pain experienced by the rats. The weight gain of the rats that consumed high fructose corn syrup may have resulted from a slowed or stalled metabolism. The weight gain may have resulted because the rats became less active and expended less energy because of fatigue, pain, or discomfort. (Or, a combination of both reasons.)

Observations and measurements of the most complicated and intricate processes of metabolism require advanced technology and sophisticated instruments. Most people do not have access to laboratories, specialized equipment, and many willing subjects.

University laboratories and research hospitals around the world are involved with many varieties of research, including studies on fibromyalgia. Reports of their results come from Great Britain, Turkey, France, and several universities throughout North America.

In recent years, interest has grown in understanding the specific and total composition of high fructose corn syrup and its effects on animals and humans. Free radicals and the browning effect are relatively new areas of research, but they appear to have relevance to the study of fibromyalgia.

The FDA has expressed concern over the chemical "fixative" used on the high fructose corn syrup mixture at the end of processing. The word "organic" is already not allowed for use on processed foods containing high fructose corn syrup. The current discussion involves a debate on whether the word "natural" is appropriate for products with high fructose corn syrup. Many believe HFCS is too synthetic and irregular to be called natural, especially since it contains unbound molecules.

Because so much is invisible to us and out of reach for our own experimentation and study, we must rely on university and college researchers and scientists in specialized fields. Important fields of study such as neuroscience, biochemistry, and endocrinology may help provide needed answers. Pain processing in the brain, activities of free radicals, and changes in the fascia appear to be particularly related to understanding fibromyalgia. The answers we have received so far are from the intellectual and medical communities in public and private institutions.

At this point, for many reasons, scientific data that answer fibromyalgia questions is sparse. Future research may yield definitive answers to the following questions:

1) What specific internal reactions are caused by monosodium glutamate?

2) What specific internal reactions are caused by aspartame?

3) What specific internal reactions are caused by the unbound molecules of high fructose corn syrup?

4) Is the unequal proportion of glucose to fructose in high fructose corn syrup a causative factor in fibromyalgia?

5) What internal processes and chemical reactions lead to the conclusion of a fibromyalgia bout?

6) Are free radicals impervious to the catalytic action of enzymes?

7) What internal processes (such as enzymes) or structures (such as intestine, membrane, or organs) allow some to have repeated episodes of fibromyalgia and others to never experience or notice any symptoms of fibromyalgia?

8) Are there any independent, unbiased scientists currently studying the long-term effects of

consuming genetically-engineered or scientifically-engineered food products?

The answers may be complex, but they are needed to support efforts by the FDA and consumer advocates. Fibromyalgia struggled to achieve legitimacy and to be acknowledged as "real" several years back. Pharmaceutical companies can count on long-term exorbitant profits as long as the public does not become aware of the root causes of fibromyalgia. Presently, independent scientists and researchers are needed to tie together all the loose ends from anecdotal reports, experiment results, medical reports, and a variety of contributions from national and international sources. Research and data collection take time, but they are important parts in the process of unveiling all definitive root causes of fibromyalgia.

Many important contributions to health and safety come from university clinics and laboratories and from thoughtful, well-versed, conscientious review by FDA scientists, and medical panels.

Chapter Fifteen

MY RECOVERY STORY

My life began in a hospital on a very cold, blustery day in Canton, Ohio. My father was serving in WWII in France. I was welcomed into the world by some nurses, my maternal grandparents and my mother. I was an imaginative, active child and a decent big sister to three siblings. I went to public schools and Sunday school. I preferred the tap dance classes over the ballet classes. Visiting with cousins was a special treat.

I spent hours playing outside with friends. On the weekend, we looked forward to a cowboy television show starring Roy Rogers. I identified heavily with Dale Evans (Roy's wife.) My brother George would stand on one side of the black and white television, and I would stand on the other side, at the close of each episode. Maybe this is corny, but we were young and innocent. We always sang the closing song with Dale and Roy. ("Happy Trails to You, Until We Meet Again . . .") Some say I had a stubborn streak, but I choose to call it tenacity.

Before the age of six, I suffered with an occasional bee sting (from playing barefoot in the yard) and from intense itchiness from poison ivy rashes. Between the ages of six and twenty, I endured two or three bouts of tonsillitis, a severe case of mumps, measles, chicken pox, several colds, and weekly piano lessons.

I was a serious child who excelled at reading, dancing, and running fast. I felt great pride when I outran all the girls in races during gym classes or when I outran my boy cousins at family reunion picnics. In short, I had no long term health crises or issues for nearly three decades. I rarely missed school during my high school years for any reason. My pregnancies, in my twenties and thirties, were relatively typical, and I gave birth with just the usual labor pains and buyer's remorse for being at the mercy of a process that was scary and took control of the lower half of my body.

In 1976 or 1977, I suffered unexplained, widespread discomfort and pain in my back and shoulders. I was confused about additional symptoms of fatigue, general achiness, and stiffness. These bouts lasted four to six days each time and came upon me eight or nine times a year. I excused the problems with a label of the flu, although the misery and chronic nature of the pain, coupled with the absence of nausea and fever, did not really match any previous experiences I had with flu. When I felt well again, I would vow to stay that way.

In the early 1980s, I knew I was not experiencing a type of influenza, and I sought medical help. The pain in my back, shoulders, and neck seemed unrelenting, at times. However, the doctor had no explanations. X-rays of my back revealed no arthritis or abnormalities in my spine. Between 1984 and 1999, I tried acupuncture, chiropractic manipulation, acupressure, aerobic classes, and psychotherapy. (I'm sure you have guessed the outcomes of those attempts.) A type of acupressure/massage was somewhat soothing to my muscles and fascia, but overall the improvement was rather minor. As optimistic as I tried to be, fibromyalgia always returned.

I researched the subject in libraries and online. I accidentally came across an article about a woman with fibromyalgia in a women's magazine. I was shocked to read about symptoms that were nearly identical to mine. I conferred with my own doctor, and he confirmed my self-diagnosis as valid. Now, I had a name for these miserable cycles. It took twelve years, but knowing a name gave me a little psychological comfort, if nothing else.

At the following doctor appointment, guaifenesin was prescribed for my daily use. Although my doctor was skeptical of its effectiveness for fibromyalgia, he said the ingredients were relatively harmless and nothing would be lost by taking it. The theory behind a guaifenesin regimen is that guiafenesin has chelating properties and its molecules will bind with the toxic molecules in the body. Then, ultimately, together the chelating agent and the toxin would be expelled from the body. We experimented for more than a year before it became apparent that this treatment was of very little value for fibromyalgia relief.

Some co-workers and friends suggested that I was high-strung and was, therefore, too sensitive to life's disappointments. A few years of psychotherapy helped free me of some emotional issues. However, the fibromyalgia continued. I learned that my bouts of fibromyalgia had no relationship to stressful times, traumatic events, or even the good, healthy exciting days of my life.

Missing work was filled with regret because I understood that most people at that time (1980s and 1990s) either had not heard of fibromyalgia or else they believed it to be basically a figment of my imagination. When I returned to work after a day or two of bed rest and very long hours of sleeping, co-workers would compliment me on how well I looked. (Irony, I guess)

I missed work between six and ten times each year, typically for one or two days. At home when I was sick, I spent most of the time, either in bed resting or curled up and sleeping fitfully hour after hour.

The stiffness and tightness in my neck, upper back and shoulders were most noticeable near the end of each fibromyalgia cycle. I would find a door jamb or corner when I could rub my back along the spinal column. My gentle son Matthew was always willing to massage my back and shoulders. My sweet daughter Amber would oblige me and walk upon my back when I laid prone on the floor. Matt and Amber willingly helped with many chores and some meal preparation. It is pleasing to me that neither of them has shown signs of fibromyalgia.

In the late 1990s, few ideas were coming from the established medical fields or from those practicing holistic healing. I searched the internet, frequently checking the primary medical websites. Advertisements for mattresses or lifting devices or liquid concoctions were sadly amusing and obviously irrelevant.

My most difficult years with fibromyalgia were from about 1981 through 2006. There was a point at which I admitted to myself that it was quite possible that I would struggle with pain, fatigue, and general misery for several days at a time for the rest of my life. I frequently prayed for relief and for answers. ("Seek and ye shall find")

From much experience, I realized that after each bout of fibromyalgia, there would be several good, pain-free days. (Maybe as long as several weeks at a time.) It was also promising that my overall health was not deteriorating, and I could keep up in dance classes with much younger dancers on good days.

My most miserable experiences were those in which I was in pain and unable to stay awake for more than an hour or two. My respiration became very shallow. During those difficult days, I felt no hunger, but I was miserable and almost felt like I had been poisoned. Spending that much time sleeping meant, of course, that I had to suspend obligations, relationships, and activities for the duration. Lower stomach cramps and diarrhea usually signaled that the cycle was coming to a very welcome end.

One morning in 2007, I was comfortably sleeping in a curled up position on my side under the covers. I was crossing the line between deep sleep and semi-consciousness. I heard a quiet voice say distinctly, "high fructose corn syrup." I realize that this is an unusual account. However, my memory and account of this occurrence are both accurate. You may explain it any way you want.

My research and study broadened to include the manufacture of high fructose corn syrup and recovery reports of others. I made records of my food intake and ate most meals at home for awhile. Reading ingredient labels became a permanent necessity in my life. When I was careless, I would know of my mistakes beginning about two or three days later.

I've made a few mistakes in food choices. A good example of an error is an occasion when I selected a small carton of cottage cheese. I had read the ingredient label of plain cottage cheese on a previous shopping trip. On this particular trip, I spotted a carton that had pineapple mixed in with it. I was in a hurry and picked up the cottage cheese with pineapple added—without reading the label. I ate most of the carton for lunch. Two days later, I felt tired and realized I was headed for a bad spell. I was confused because I remembered, at that time, very careful food choices. Pain set in by day three or four. By day four or five, my neck and shoulders were very tight, and I could hear crackling noises when I turned my head to look to the right or left. Eventually, I recalled the cottage cheese purchase. On my next grocery trip, I found the same brand and read the label and discovered the dairy had added high fructose corn syrup into the cottage cheese.

By reading ingredient labels, carefully preparing food, and being highly selective when I eat out, I have been successful at preventing fibromyalgia symptoms. The dramatic difference in my life is literally "awesome." I am grateful everyday and hope that others will have similar experiences with successful recovery. It is regrettable that I had so many years of struggling, and I lost many days and hours of energy and full engagement with many activities. However, fibromyalgia is behind me now. My recovery is a blessing that I will never take for granted.

It is very satisfying knowing that I have never taken fibromyalgia medications with disclaimers that suggest potential serious side effects, such as breathing difficulties, weight gain, blisters or hives, unusual behavior or mood changes, or soreness and muscle pain.

My natural method is healthy and does not bring about any thoughts of suicide. (Many prescription medications currently advertised warn of suicidal thoughts as one of the potential side effects of the medication.) Without fibromyalgia, I have more energy, time, strength, and overall contentment.

CHAPTER SIXTEEN

GOOD HEALTH

The overall health of the total U.S. population has been declining in the last couple of decades. According to reports from 2010, health in the United States has earned lower ratings than the health ratings of several European and Asian countries. Poorer health for many American consumers is attributed to increases in Type 2 diabetes, obesity, Alzheimer's, heart disease and some types of cancer. Other factors are the high cost of health care in the United States and the lack of care for the poorest citizens.

Many are surprised to learn that the U.S. is also surpassed by several countries on measures of longevity (average life span). There are several reasons that help account for a average shorter life span in the U.S. than in other countries. Much of the population travels regularly by car. In 2010, more than 32,000 Americans died in traffic accidents on roads and freeways.

For reasons unknown or for reasons not yet published, infant mortality rates in the U.S. have been high for a long time. Rates of alcoholism are higher in the U.S. than in several other countries. Also, there are serious health conditions and deaths that result from dependence on illegal drugs and from legal, prescribed medications. Death can result from overdoses of drugs, whether or not the drug is legal or illegal.

Another factor that contributes to a lower rank on longevity scales is the ever-growing number of "homeless" citizens who take up residence in cars, subways, or under freeway passes. The street people in the U.S. cities are a combination of mentally ill, disenfranchised citizens, substance addicts, run-aways, and victims of a long-term, serious economic downturn. In the last three decades, millions of jobs have been replaced with computers or relocated to countries that compensate workers at much lower levels of pay than the U.S. minimum wage. Obviously, one dollar an hour for production is much more attractive to manufacturers than eight or nine dollars an hour. Many jobs in Mexico and India pay less than a dollar an hour for work. In many other countries, including Mexico and India, benefits such as overtime compensation, vacation pay, or illness pay exist for only a few. Therefore, companies who relocate in other countries pay significantly less in wages and for all other forms of work compensation.

Many people in American survive on very small incomes. Those who live without pay and compensation for months or years slip deeply into poverty, debt, and homelessness. A recent report revealed that the average age of death for a transient or a long-term street person is a little over 59 years. Their shorter lives are attributed to the lack of medical care, unsanitary living conditions, poor diets, and physical risks, especially for those who live in an environment of drug and human trafficking.

It is believed that if statistics from infant mortality, fatal traffic accidents, as well as transient death rates, were excluded from computations, the United States would fare much better on longevity comparisons. (Of course, rather than manipulating the statistics, it would be better to find ways to reduce traffic accidents, reduce the number of infant deaths, and address socio-economic conditions that play heavily into job loss and home loss.)

More Americans die each year from cancer than from any other cause. For several years in a row, the fatality rate for cancer in the United States has remained at a number considerably higher than 500,000. Lung cancer deaths have declined somewhat, but deaths from most types of cancer have continued to increase. Some preliminary research has linked some cancer growth with some food additives, especially chemical, man-made additives. (Of course, carcinogens are in many substances, natural and unnatural, and in non-food substances in the environment.) It is impossible to avoid all substances that are classified as carcinogens.

Most of us hope for a long life with good health, vibrancy, mobility, and optimism. We are not in control of all of life's circumstances. However, most of us are fortunate enough to enjoy the protection of a home and receive an income that allows for regular purchase of quality groceries and food. We can choose healthy products. Last year, more than a thousand new grocery products were stocked in stores. Some contribute to good health, some are called "empty calories" (without nutrients), and some contain ingredients which have the potential to do harm.

You have learned that many processed foods contain chemical ingredients or foods whose basic DNA have been changed (denatured). These ingredients are the primary causes of the symptoms you experience with fibromyalgia. Read all ingredient labels and select and order food carefully.

Completely omit all high fructose corn syrup in beverages and foods for six to eight weeks (Plan A). After eight weeks you should feel and experience much less pain, stiffness and fatigue. If you are more than eighty percent recovered after eight weeks, it is safe to assume that high fructose corn syrup is the toxic substance most responsible for your problems. You will continue to improve as long as you omit all HFCS.

If Plan A is barely providing relief for you and you are still experiencing all-over pain and chronic fatigue, you have a more chronic type of fibromyalgia. The most severe types of fibromyalgia are probably caused by several xenobiotics. Recovery will require eliminating as many xenobiotics and man-made chemicals as possible. Research has not yet identified all chemicals that are harmful to some with fibromyalgia. Therefore, eliminating as many xenobiotics as possible should provide relief. If you have not been successful with Plan A, begin Plan B. (Both plans are detailed in Chapter Two of this book.) Restrict your diet to only organic food and carefully follow the guidelines detailed in Plan B. Anecdotal accounts from reliable sources point to monosodium glutamate (MSG) and aspartame (artificial sweetener) as fibromyalgia causes.

Recent reports state that all artificial sweeteners, including sucralose, can compromise health with long-term use. Using natural sweeteners is preferable. Limiting the use of artificial sweeteners or avoiding them completely is a wise habit to develop.

I read all ingredient labels, at least before purchasing the product the first time. I carefully avoid all products that contain high fructose corn syrup. In addition, I drink organic milk (milk without added hormones). I suspect that some of the hormones that effect the mammary glands of cows (added to increase milk production) probably have the potential to effect human mammary glands also. I meticulously follow Plan A to maintain a relatively pain-free existence. I also avoid MSG and aspartame, but not with the same level of commitment and ingredient scrutiny that I employ for avoiding high fructose corn syrup.

In the past decade, scientists have emphasized the importance of greatly limiting trans fats in the diet. American manufacturers are required to print the amount of trans fats on the product label. There is some debate over saturated fats, but most nutritionists advise consumers to use saturated fats sparingly. Healthy fats are those in avocados, peanuts, seeds, olives, coconuts, and all varieties of tree nuts. (All of those fats are "real" foods.) Olive oil is a nutritious, tasty choice to use when blending a salad dressing or making a dip.

Most of us have easy access to a great variety of packaged breads. Remember that whole grains are significantly higher in nutrients and fiber than white bread. Whole wheat bread is preferable to white bread, but it is not quite as nutritious as whole grain breads.

The average American diet contains too much sodium, sugar, and fat. If anything is lacking in your diet, it can probably be gained by eating nuts, beans, fish, meats, vegetables, seeds, or fruits. Eating a wide variety of fruits and vegetables will ultimately strengthen your immune system, add fiber to your diet, and provide important vitamins and minerals. Your doctor may recommend dietary supplements. Some nutritionists suggest that people with fibromyalgia use Vitamin D and magnesium supplements.

A daily dose of sunlight exposure of at least twenty minutes in length is advisable. If that is not feasible, ask your doctor to recommend an appropriate dosage level of a vitamin D supplement. Indoor dogs and cats seek out a sunny spot to rest or nap frequently. Animals seem to have great intuition, or maybe they enjoy the warmth of the sun.

In an earlier book, I advised people to avoid eating rice because of high arsenic levels—well above the recommended level of the FDA. Twelve to fifteen years ago, scientific measurements of the levels of arsenic in American rice yielded alarming results.

Some believed the high arsenic content in rice was caused by treatments sprayed on American crops of cotton decades ago. During the time of cotton crops, very strong pesticides were used to kill boll weevils. Boll weevils on cotton crops threatened the livelihood of cotton farmers, if the boll weevils were not destroyed in time. The pesticides contained arsenic. Years later, rice was planted in the same fields that once grew cotton. The soil was still saturated with arsenic. As the rice grew, many believe, it absorbed the arsenic from the soil.

For several reasons, I no longer have concerns about the safety of rice. I have found no detrimental reports about rice in recent years. Over the past ten years, many rice fields have been flooded several times, allowing for the dilution of any remaining arsenic. In addition, many rice products are imported from other parts of the world. Rice is an important and nutritious staple in many diets.

Antioxidants are molecules in certain foods that have the potential to slow oxidation in the body. Selecting foods that add antioxidants to the diet is being emphasized more frequently by health professionals. Antioxidants are molecules found in fruits and vegetables which can counter some of the negative effects of free radicals. It is believed that in addition to improving overall health, antioxidants help protect eyesight and mitigate some of the environmental factors that contribute to aging.

A general rule for selecting high level antioxidant fruits and vegetables it to select the ones with the deepest and most vibrant colors. Excellent choices are blueberries, kale, parsley, cilantro, raspberries, blackberries, pecans, walnuts, beets, dried kidney beans, pinto beans, prunes, cranberries, artichoke hearts, and turmeric.

Walking, aerobic exercise, bicycling, swimming, and other forms of exercise benefit the brain and the body. Increasing oxygen consumption through exercise, qigong, or deep breathing relaxes the body and provides greater amounts of oxygen. An experienced M.D. was questioned regarding his expert opinion on what one change the average American could make to improve his or her health. The doctor answered that several minutes of deep breathing exercises done on a daily basis would contribute to an improvement in overall health.

The importance of getting adequate sleep should not be ignored. For many, family and home recreation and responsibilities, including time spent watching television, operating computers, and communicating with hand-held devices, are devouring huge portions of each day. Many have extensive job requirements with project deadlines. Others have class assignments to complete in the evening. Our demanding, busy lives leave an insufficient amount of time for sleep. Good health requires an adequate amount of restorative sleep time.

If you are still suffering with fibromyalgia, then you do not have regular control over sleep patterns. Your sleep may remain fitful until you have become victorious over fibromyalgia.

Most adults benefit from seven to nine hours of sleep each day. When you are relaxed and in the stage of deep sleep, important repair functions are performed internally—on the skin, in the cells, and some say, in the mind.

Many say, "Good health is everything!" Good health is a requirement for the fullest participation in life. It ranks at the top of the list with love and laughter.

CHAPTER SEVENTEEN

HAPPY ENDING

We have much to be grateful for. If your recovery is already in progress, I am sure you share my gratitude and optimism. Although this book is not long, it contains quite a bit of information. Below is a summary of some of the critical points:

- Almost every condition and disease has a cure. Finding the root cause is the first step in developing an effective cure. If treatments are limited to SYMPTOM control, then the basic problem and the need for treatment might continue throughout one's whole life.

- Fibromyalgia did not exist prior to 1970—not the name, not the particular set of symptoms, and not as an existing medical classification with a different name. Fibromyalgia is relatively new. Reports of the new, unique widespread pain syndrome began in the 1970s. Fibromyalgia was given its name in the early 1980s.

- A label of "organic" means the food product meets the FDA standards of quality and contains only natural ingredients.

- Honest research results are reported by independent, non-profit laboratories. Representatives from companies with financial interests in potential products are too biased to be forthcoming and reliable and often present only the data that supports their interests.

- Universities, agencies, and researchers that value truth and welfare and fair treatment of all citizens deserve appreciation and support. Healthy bodies, sound minds and credible sources of information work together to protect democracy.

- The root causes of fibromyalgia are man-made chemicals infused into processed foods. After consumption, these unnatural additives negatively affect the basic elements of metabolism (cellular, enzyme, and neurotransmitter activities). Nerves are a part of metabolism, too. However, "nerves" are not, and never have been, the root cause of fibromyalgia.

- Remember to read all ingredient labels prior to purchasing, unless the container states that the product is "organic."

- High fructose corn syrup is a manufactured, denatured substance used in processed foods. Because of the unusually long lull between consumption of HFCS and its unfortunate effects, many overlook the cause and effect relationship.

- Corn sugar, high fructose corn syrup and HFCS are all the same manufactured substance!

Consumers have organized into groups that lobby for safe food products and clear, truthful labeling on ingredient labels. Universities around the world are leading the way on research of real causes and real cures for many medical issues, including fibromyalgia. Researchers at Princeton University have provided an important research stepping stone by sharing the results of the experiments on high fructose corn syrup.

Many manufacturers are using alternative sweeteners in place of high fructose corn syrup. Consumer groups have organized their efforts to convince the FDA that MSG, aspartame, and high fructose corn syrup should not be designated as "GRAS." FDA approval should be reserved for only those chemicals that are above the suspicion of scientists and have proven records of safety.

The medical world and the larger society no longer view us as sensitive personalities or as victims of our own over-active imaginations. In the last few decades, fibromyalgia has been upgraded from a psychosomatic syndrome or a mystery condition to a legitimate biochemical disorder.

Canaries were used by coal miners before the regular use of measurement instruments. The borrowed analogy seems fitting. Those with fibromyalgia are sensitive to toxins in the environment as canaries are sensitive to poisonous fumes in mines. Prior to entering a suspicious mine area, miners placed canaries. If the canaries died, then miners knew that they might die also if they breathed the same air. Similarly, those with fibromyalgia appear to react to toxins in food and water before the general population. Unlike the caged canaries, we have many options.

We have the knowledge and power to make wise food and beverage selections. Most of us have the resources to be selective, and we have access to a great variety of healthy foods. Prevention is the key for fibromyalgia. "An ounce of prevention is worth a pound of cure."

I am especially grateful for a recovery regimen that is natural and gentle and does not subject my body to potent drugs that bring with them warnings and a long list of potential side effects. In addition to living without pain, stiffness and periodic chronic fatigue, I know I am protecting my health. In addition, I avoid the expense of long-term prescription medications.

If you exclude high fructose corn syrup completely and reduce the amount of man-made chemicals in your diet, you will experience renewed energy and much less pain and stiffness. You will have energy for work and relationships. In addition to being free of most fibromyalgia symptoms, it is likely your overall health will improve.

I am happy that my long struggle with fibromyalgia is over, and I have been freed from unnecessary pain, discomfort, and limitation. My work on this book is almost complete. I'm looking forward to seeing more movies, reading more books, and living vicariously through my grandchildren.

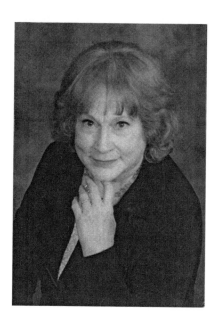

Janice Lorigan is a researcher, analyst and grandmother who lives in southern California. During her career, she lived and worked in Washington, D.C., Ohio, Virginia and California. She received B.A. and M.A. degrees in Psychology from California State University, Los Angeles.

Our author enjoys traveling, movies, and reading. She feels passionate about fairness and safety for consumers, democratic representation for everyone, and maintaining a nation that values education, human rights and fair compensation for labor

CPSIA information can be obtained at www.ICGtesting.com
Printed in the USA
241565LV00001B/131/P

9 781463 407865